Sudden Death

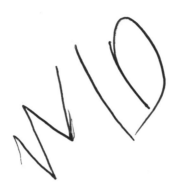

For *Churchill Livingstone:*

Commissioning editor: Inta Ozols/ Alex Mathieson
Project development editor: Valerie Bain
Project manager: Valerie Burgess
Project controller: Derek Robertson
Design direction: Judith Wright
Copy editor: Sarah Firman
Indexer: Nina Boyd
Sales promotion executive: Hilary Brown

Sudden Death

A Research Base for Practice

Bob Wright Hon MSc RGN RMN
Clinical Nurse Specialist (Crisis Care), Accident & Emergency Department,
Leeds General Infirmary, Leeds, UK

SECOND EDITON

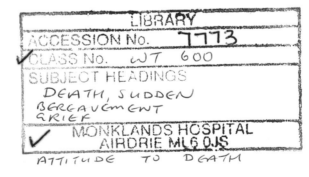
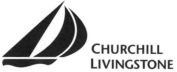

CHURCHILL
LIVINGSTONE

EDINBURGH, LONDON, NEW YORK, PHILADELPHIA, ST LOUIS, SYDNEY, TORONTO 1996

CHURCHILL LIVINGSTONE
An imprint of Harcourt Publishers Limited

⬧ is a registered trademark of Harcourt Publishers Limited

© Pearson Professional Limited
© Harcourt Publishers Limited 1999

First published 1991
  Reprinted 1993
Second edition 1996
  Reprinted 1999

ISBN 0 443 05459 2

British Library of Cataloguing in Publication Data
A catalogue record for this book is available from the British Library.

Library of Congress Cataloging in Publication Data
A catalogue record for this book is available from the Library of Congress.

The
publisher's
policy is to use
**paper manufactured
from sustainable forests**

Printed in China

Contents

Preface to second edition

It is 5 years since this book was first published. During that time my work and involvement in this area has grown. As a full-time Clinical Nurse Specialist in Crisis Care, the major part of my work involves sudden death and trauma. The resulting grief and post-traumatic stress has required many hours of counselling as well as work at the time of impact. The counselling of children has increased, and so I have now included a chapter on caring for the suddenly bereaved child. The other changes in the book reflect my continuing experiences of counselling the suddenly bereaved, caring for the staff, and teaching and training.

The teaching and training makes up one-third of my role and involves many disciplines. In multidisciplinary training sessions, both I and the participants are consoled by the knowledge that the difficulties with this kind of work are common to us all. Members of the police, fire and ambulance services, as well as nurses, social workers, doctors, counsellors, teachers and chaplaincy workers, all admit to experiencing periods of vulnerability. How we encounter death may differ, but we all share the way it highlights our human frailty.

From training these people (as members of organizations or as multidisciplinary groups), it is obvious that we need all the help we can get. Debriefing disastrous and critical incidents has taught me a great deal about the strengths and the philosophies of many of these workers. It has also revealed how the workers' fundamental beliefs are challenged and how resources at all levels are demanded. Preparing, teaching, training and supporting the personnel remains an essential part of this book.

Listening daily to stories of sudden and traumatic deaths, which I do as nurse and counsellor, could take its toll. The staff in the Accident & Emergency department care for me, and I value this. I am provided with on-going supervision which, along with the support of my wife, children, family and friends, serves to remind me of the things that are valuable in life.

I must emphasize that I also gain from my clients and my work. The many examples used in this book will show that our clients have much to teach us. They all, including the children, tell stories of pain, distress and profound sadness. They also demonstrate courage, wisdom and the determination to survive against all odds. 'What could be so disruptive, so ravaging and cruel, and so utterly out of control that could change our lives in such a way, that life as we knew it could never be the same again' (Gregory 1995). As this grieving mother shows in her description, sudden death is an outrage. Words cannot do justice to the pain experienced in every dimension of the person.

Since the first edition of this book, most change has taken place in our response to sudden death and our knowledge of people's needs. More information on caring at the time of impact, and on the response of the organization, can now be included.

The theoretical framework of crisis intervention underpins some of our personal response. Completely new to this edition are my thoughts on listening to the wholly personal experience of the sudden death. Listening is a major part of my work, not only at the time of impact but also during the difficult journey through the grief. Much more attention is given to listening to and hearing the story; it is an essential part of the healing process and of re-emergence from being overwhelmed with pain.

The particular difficulties involved in the death of a child are now given a separate chapter.

This second edition reflects my daily experiences with the suddenly bereaved as well as the work of others who have influenced my knowledge and practice. References to 'our' study identify the work of Marjorie Ashdown and myself in which we evaluated the care of 100 suddenly bereaved relatives. This looked at their response at the impact of the death at the hospital, the care they received, and the difficulties experienced by the worker. Staff involved were interviewed within 1 or 2 days about their perception of the event. The bereaved relatives were seen between 6 and 10 months after the death, to discover their perception of the care they received.

One criticism of our study is that the methodology is unclear (McDonald et al 1995). The information obtained from staff and bereaved relatives can best be described as qualitative. Much of the material is descriptive of situations and events. Material from each interview with staff and relatives was organized under headings and subheadings. Brief notes were made telling the story of each case. A comparison of these stories revealed interesting patterns and responses. I appreciate, however, that the influence of the researchers in the construction of the data should be taken into account. Qualitative comparative analysis or grounded theory, as described by Glaser & Strauss (1967), is important for theory development. The theory then needs to be tested, using a more formal approach to validate it.

For student readers, activities to help reinforce the ideas presented are included in each chapter. I hope these will also discourage readers from being passive recipients of information, and help them to feel more involved in the discussion.

This revised edition describes, I hope, the more enlightened care of the suddenly bereaved and their carers which has evolved since the first edition. My other hope is that my enthusiasm for the work, and for the search for further insights and knowledge, are also reflected in this book.

Leeds 1996   B. W.

REFERENCES

Glaser B, Strauss A 1967 The discovery of grounded theory: strategies for qualitative research. Aldene Publishing, Chicago
Gregory C M 1995 I should have been with Lisa as she died. Journal of Accident & Emergency Nursing 3(3): 136–138
McDonald L, Butterworth T, Yates D W 1995 Grief support in Accident & Emergency nursing: a literature review 1985–1993. Journal of Accident & Emergency Nursing 3(3): 154–157

Acknowledgements

First, thanks are due to my wife, children and family for their listening and encouragement, and their support of my work, which is intrusive by nature.

Marjorie Ashdown was not only deeply involved with the study, but also continues to work closely with me, debriefing disastrous events and critical incidents, and in many training sessions. Her insight, support and friendship and sense of humour are important to me.

My clients and their families are a source of knowledge, strength and inspiration to me. They generously gave permission to use the whole or part of their stories in this book.

I know I belong to and am supported by my colleagues at Leeds General Infirmary, especially in the Accident & Emergency Department. They are a special group of people to whom I am indebted.

Finally, Anne Jacques spends many hours not only reading my writing but sorting out problems and mistakes to produce the final draft for the publishers. Hers is the skill that makes more sense of it for you and corrects my English, and liaises with the publishers whose great help is also valued.

1

The crisis of sudden death

Sudden death is well recognized as one of the most traumatic crisis events that can be experienced. How we begin to work with this will be explained in more detail later. First, it is helpful to have some understanding of the studies which have been made into crisis intervention. This approach can clarify some of the difficulties as they arise and provide a greater sense of the overall management of the crisis.

However, this background information should not prevent healthcare professionals from engaging with the immediate dynamics of the situation. Some of these interactions will be painful and distressing for workers. It is important to realize that the professional's responses are a valuable part of the process of the crisis and of the longer process of grief for the client. Those who come into contact with these crisis clients and work with them, need to know that despite the difficulties they themselves experience, the work is worthwhile.

All the evidence shows that sudden death can be damaging and disabling to those bereaved (Lindemann 1944, Bowlby 1981, Lundin 1984, Murphy 1988). The absence of an opportunity to anticipate the grief was first discussed in Lindemann's paper which is now considered a classic. Lindemann's contribution to the theory of crisis intervention is based on the Coconut Grove (night club) fire of 1944. The study found that the fire resulted in a crisis for all individuals closely involved and demonstrated that interventionists need not take control of the individual affected, but rather help him to move into a normal coping process.

Lindemann's approach to crisis intervention was described in more depth by Caplan (1964). Caplan's theories about life crisis acknowledged Erikson's (1950) model of developmental (maturational) and situational (accidental) crisis (see Table 1.1).

Table 1.1   Situational and developmental crisis

Situational (accidental)	Developmental (maturational)
Sudden illness	Birth
Accident	Puberty/adolescence
Redundancy	Courtship
Loss of income	Marriage
Loss of status	Pregnancy
Loss of security	Menopause
Divorce/separation	Death

Caplan described developmental crisis as transitional periods in personality development, characterized by disturbances in affective and cognitive functioning. A sudden unexpected threat to, or loss of, basic resources or life goals constitutes a situational crisis.

Situational crises, which form the majority of my work, can lead to intensive periods of psychological, behavioural and physical disarray. Caplan observed that situational crises are often new to the client and that their usual coping methods do not work.

Some crises may be compounded by fitting into both categories. A 20-year-old woman, for example, may, within a month of her marriage, suffer the death of her husband in a road traffic accident. A developmental crisis, her marriage, is compounded by a situational crisis, the accident, which has the power to throw her life into disarray. We cannot treat her loss, and the emotionally painful experience of the loss, without discussing the distress of all this happening within a month of her marriage.

Whilst this example identifies clearly the two types of crisis, others may not be so easily identified. We need to be aware of where the client is on the developmental scale (life's milestones), in order to appreciate fully the implications of a sudden death. Placing a client's experience of loss on his life milestone graph (Fig. 1.1), noting the stage he is now at, or may be heading towards or leaving, is a useful exercise. Further discussion with the client about his perception of his life situation may alter assumptions we have made about him.

Some situational crises, such as redundancy, divorce or separation, produce a loss of status and security. Again, if these are marked along the line of life's developmental crises, their overwhelming nature may be perceived. Caplan (1964) says that even individuals with relatively stable personalities can change in unexpected ways during such a crisis.

Activity 1A

Pick one life crisis from the maturational list and one from the situational list (Table 1.1). Describe which one may be the most difficult to manage, and explain why.

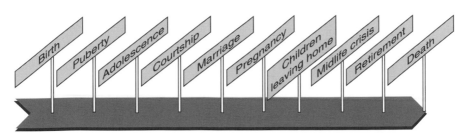

Figure 1.1   Life's milestones.

The change needed to deal with crisis may have positive aspects, highlighting the opportunities that crisis can bring. On the other hand, the crisis can result in an increased inability to cope, and lead to feelings of chaos and disorder. This leads to the view that a crisis is a transitional period offering the individual an opportunity for growth or increasing their vulnerability.

Time is another aspect to consider. A crisis cannot be tolerated for a long period because it involves intense feelings of distress and disorder which have the capacity to damage. Carers not only have to respond quickly but, as discussed later in this book, frequent and lengthy periods of care will also be necessary in order to prevent damage and restore equilibrium.

Caplan viewed crisis intervention as a major part of preventive psychiatry. He believed that individuals could be supported and offered the right conditions to deal effectively with crisis, thereby preventing mental disorder.

This book attempts to explore the wider implications of sudden death, from its impact through to coping with the loss. Crisis intervention, I believe, offers us a place to begin the process of dealing with loss. Opportunities taken at the time of the sudden death are crucial in determining the ability of the bereaved person to accept and cope with the crisis (Dubin & Sarnoff 1986, Fraser & Atkins 1990).

The importance of reassuring and affirming a person's feelings, from the moment of impact through on-going support, in healing the grief was recognized by Rogers & Reich (1988). The crisis model shown in Fig. 1.2 provides a useful framework for intervention. It identifies three routes to explore when dealing with the crisis of sudden death, as outlined next.

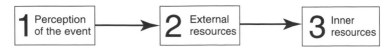

Figure 1.2   Three routes to explore when attempting to cope with crisis.

1. The client's *perception of the event* influences how he is able to face the reality of the situation. It is important to ask him to describe the event and what it means to him, in terms of his plans, his hopes, his aspirations. How the event changes his life, the present and the future need to be discussed. The client's realistic appraisal of the event is essential. Its impact and the likelihood of disorder to follow are very apparent at this stage. The client will usually mention that self-esteem is damaged; what we mean by self-esteem will be examined in more detail later.

2. *External resources* available to help the client cope with this event are the second factor to work with. The disordered activity resulting from the impact of the event often makes it difficult for the client to think logically about sources of strength, comfort and support, and may actually prevent him from accessing them. The first resources to explore are usually family and friends, or other people close to the client and on intimate terms with him. The person in crisis knows his need of them but the disarray and distress produce fear that he will not reach them. This may be expressed clearly as: 'Please help me find my brother, he will help me, he will know what to do.' This expectation of the help to be received may well be unrealistic initially, but as time progresses, and with help, more order will replace disorder.

The external resources may also include other disciplines, caring agencies and organizations or self-help groups. It is important to be aware of local resources and the types of help available.

3. The client may be able to access *inner resources* in coping with a crisis. He should be helped to realize his strengths and vulnerabilities. The overwhelming feeling at a time of crisis is that any forward movement is impossible; the client is rendered impotent and this increases his distress. The fear produced by being immobilized is tremendously powerful; it can make one feel totally weak, or lead to panic.

Acknowledging inner strengths and feelings can result in activity and movement forward, enhancing potency or effectiveness. This feels positive and suggests some advance towards management of the problem. It is important for the client's self-esteem that he can ask 'What can I do about this?' and begin to look at answers and alternatives for himself.

If we can help the client to look at and work positively with these three aspects of coping with a stressful event — perception of the event, external resources, inner resources — a crisis may be averted. Perception of the event will have a strong negative content if there is denial of the meaning or the reality of the situation. Negative responses will also arise if external resources are poor or not available. The client's inability to access resources, strengths or insights within himself will make exploration of the third area a non-productive exercise. One or two negative responses in these areas are likely to lead to a life crisis if the client's position remains unchanged.

A client's failure to find a way of working with his problems may be due to his refusing to acknowledge or explore these three areas previously mentioned, and it may be necessary to keep returning to them. He may not be motivated towards a resolution in any case. Helpers must be aware that they do not control outcomes and cannot always achieve success, whatever this means to each client. The ultimate success or outcome of an intervention lies with the client, and not with those helping.

Helpers will encounter problems if they try to seek a quick conclusion to crisis intervention. A sense of the real value of this work will help with any concern about time commitment. The initiative in helping someone to begin work on his crisis is important. The client may feel able to reveal previously unspoken thoughts to a helper at this time. This may give the helper insights into the many powerful emotional difficulties that could prevent the start of recovery and will require the concentrated, motivated effort of the client to overcome.

THE FOUR PHASES OF CRISIS

There are four recognized phases of crisis (see Fig. 1.3), although individuals do not necessarily experience all phases. Using the three routes described earlier to explore ways of coping when confronted with crisis can enable the client to leave the process, i.e. begin to manage the crisis, before reaching the severe stage.

However, this is not a magic formula. In sudden death there is no quick answer, but we can help clients to *begin* the process of managing their feelings of chaos and disorder.

STATUS

A sudden death can instantly or more insidiously damage a person's status. By status I mean the position or standing in society which governs the respect or rights people receive. Their status may give them a role or a place, somewhere they belong. If this is suddenly removed it leaves them vulnerable or seeking a new status:

'Where do I stand now?'
'Does this relate to what I thought I had?'
'This is like starting all over again.'

Some people describe having to make a completely new start or an about turn after a crisis. Image and status can be closely bound together.

Activity 1B

Describe a sequence of events leading to a crisis situation.

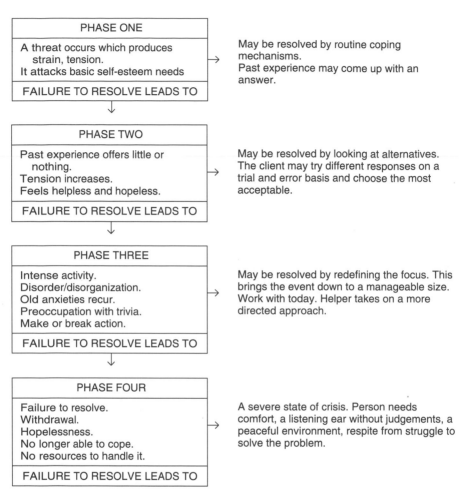

PHASE ONE	
A threat occurs which produces strain, tension. It attacks basic self-esteem needs	→ May be resolved by routine coping mechanisms. Past experience may come up with an answer.
FAILURE TO RESOLVE LEADS TO	

↓

PHASE TWO	
Past experience offers little or nothing. Tension increases. Feels helpless and hopeless.	→ May be resolved by looking at alternatives. The client may try different responses on a trial and error basis and choose the most acceptable.
FAILURE TO RESOLVE LEADS TO	

↓

PHASE THREE	
Intense activity. Disorder/disorganization. Old anxieties recur. Preoccupation with trivia. Make or break action.	→ May be resolved by redefining the focus. This brings the event down to a manageable size. Work with today. Helper takes on a more directed approach.
FAILURE TO RESOLVE LEADS TO	

↓

PHASE FOUR	
Failure to resolve. Withdrawal. Hopelessness. No longer able to cope. No resources to handle it.	→ A severe state of crisis. Person needs comfort, a listening ear without judgements, a peaceful environment, respite from struggle to solve the problem.
FAILURE TO RESOLVE LEADS TO	

Figure 1.3 The phases of crisis.

We have discussed how a client's place along the life's milestones graph may indicate a developmental crisis; it may also highlight a threat to the client's status. For example, a shift towards retirement or a mother's children growing up and leaving home, or the end of a woman's sexually reproductive period, indicates a new role and a change in status.

THE DETERMINANTS OF GRIEF

In his 1975 study, Parkes identified determinants or predictors of grief. These are factors in a death that determine difficulties in working towards a satisfactory outcome. I tend to avoid using the word 'resolution' in crisis work. One question I have often been asked is:

'Is grief ever resolved?'

It may be more realistic to say that one works — or struggles — towards living with this loss.

The determinants of grief identified in Parkes' study are as follows:

- mode of death
- nature of the attachment
- who was the person?
- historical antecedents
- personality variables
- social variables.

Some observations about these determinants from my own experience of counselling people who have suffered a sudden death follow here. Over my years in acute psychiatry, counselling and critical care nursing I have discovered the value of identifying these determinants. They pinpoint difficulties which become recurring issues in counselling. If they are borne in mind when you listen to a client's account of the loss, you will be aware of the part these components play in his reaction to the crisis.

They may be dealt with quickly or trivialized because the client feels intense pain when considering them. A helper may need to return to the painful area later and an awareness of the determinants helps with this.

Mode of death

If the death was from 'natural causes' such as an illness, even if it was sudden, it is likely to cause fewer problems than traumatic death. Death by injury, which damages the body, is more likely to be thought of as causing suffering and as being an injustice.

Most people will ask whether the deceased suffered or knew anything about the act or process of dying. It will be more difficult to blame others if the death was due to illness, but they may blame themselves for not having the foresight to call a doctor or an ambulance sooner. The professional ability or resources of individuals in the Health Service may be blamed. Much time and effort will be needed to explore the issues around this.

Death by road traffic accident, or accident at work or at home, can cause anger and a sense of injustice far greater than does natural sudden death. Things are even worse when monetary compensation is an issue — this usually falls short in that it somehow devalues the deceased.

The verdict of the Coroner's Court or finding of the Fatal Accident Inquiry is often discussed at length, as is the question of whether the deceased was entirely blameless in relation to his own death. If the deceased was not to blame, something or some person is usually felt to be responsible. The area of responsibility may be even wider — if a person or organization was not to blame, then culture or society may be blamed. In some extremes, civilization or mankind is blamed and the bereaved person may isolate himself from society, resulting in an even greater loss.

John's parents believed that the importance attached locally to traffic and commuters resulted in or contributed to their son's death. Commuters parked on both sides of the road on every working day: there was no car park despite local pressure for one. As a result, the road was narrow and its curve also caused problems, particularly for heavy goods vehicles.

John and his friend died instantly when John's motorbike was struck by a lorry. They were thrown into a wall and sustained multiple injuries. There was evidence that they had been driving too fast, although this was disputed. What was not disputed by any witnesses, including the lorry driver, was that the lorry had had to cross the centre of the road because of parked vehicles.

The official verdict was accidental death. Recommendations were made about parking restrictions. John's parents were pleased about this but who allowed it in the first place? Why does everyone need a car? Perhaps they should sell their car to make the point that cars are destroying the environment.

Over a period of months, much of their grief was worked through well. The anger and its power were diminished. Their resentment of the city's traffic policy, and how they were surrounded by it, were a constant reminder of their belief that society values people less than cars.

Eventually they moved house which resulted in further losses. Despite this, living in the country gave them some tranquillity and less ammunition for their anger and frustration about the destructive effects of traffic.

The place where a death occurred becomes an integral part of the grief. Was the deceased on home ground or in a strange place? The pain will be greater if he was far away from home. He was all alone when he died. No person around will have known him and this underlines a recurring theme that he was someone special, a big, important part of their lives. Away, he was a stranger, no one knew him, he was anonymous, alone. His real identity, the person he was, was not apparent.

That many families are now scattered throughout the world presents an added dimension to grief. This is particularly difficult if friends and neighbours did not know the deceased.

Mary received a telegram to say her brother in Australia had died suddenly. He was her only brother. He had emigrated 20 years previously, and when Mary's neighbour came to comfort her she attempted to reduce the enormity of the loss by reference to this: 'Well, never mind, you lost him a long time ago, in a sense. You couldn't be close after all this time.'

Mary kept her sadness to herself after that. Her guilt at not making the effort to visit him would remain hers. No one here knew him, they had no sense of his love, his warmth, his happy personality.

The carers, friends, neighbours and family may be at a disadvantage in having no sense of who the person was. It can reduce their ability to understand and empathize.

One mode of death that produces some tremendous difficulties is suicide. The process of grieving becomes very complicated both emotionally and intellectually. The bereaved are not only sorting out their own loss but speculating about how the victim might have emerged from his difficulty if he had remained alive. They may come up with actions that would have prevented the suicide, and this holds the potential for profound guilt.

In counselling, the one thing really valued is a chance to express powerful, ambivalent feelings. Anyone closely touched by suicide will be in need of some counselling.

Nature of the attachment

The strengths of the relationship, what its loss represents, and the security or aspects of safety gained from the relationship, are useful areas to explore because they highlight vulnerability.

One feeling that recurs in crisis is ambivalence, giving rise to much heart ache and soul searching. If there was ambivalence in the living relationship, it will certainly occur at the death and in the long term. The difficulty lies in the strong sense that this feeling is inappropriate in grief — much time can be spent in encouraging the expression of ambivalence.

Who was the person?

Who the deceased was in relation to the bereaved person must be ascertained. The deceased's position in the hierarchy of the family is not necessarily a clue to the enormity of the loss and we must not make assumptions. I can still remember talking to and trying to comfort the lover of a middle-aged man, whilst his wife sat in a room a few doors away saying she was now free to get on with her own life. Not only is the family relationship an issue, but how would you feel if your husband died at the home of his lover?

Historical antecedents

A previous life crisis, particularly a sudden death, will present as a major factor in coping. If I have experienced a previous life crisis with a good or reasonable outcome, then in theory this should help me. I will have programmed into my head something that identifies difficulty but removes or diminishes some fear about the outcome. This may be useful, provided I can get in touch with the previous experience. However, if the previous outcome was one of pain and suffering, the present problems are compounded. Previously unresolved loss or failure to confront loss may result in its re-emergence causing difficulty for the helper in establishing the focus of the loss.

Other recent life changes, crises, or recent depressive illness will result in more difficulty in handling the loss. Energy and resources used up in tackling these will have left the person drained or depleted of resources.

Personality variables

My own counselling experience shows that personality affects the search for a healthy resolution to grief. Positive coping with the immediate grief does not guarantee a lack of long-term problems. The personality that allows self-actualization, a feeling of some control over one's own life, and sees problems as a challenge seems to be most likely to recover.

Raphael (1984) writes that, although no specific risk factors have been demonstrated, certain personal characteristics may carry a risk of poor outcome. These include ambivalence and dependent or clinging relationships.

Earlier personal experience of grief, especially childhood loss of parent/s, contributes to vulnerability. I have witnessed this re-emerging vulnerability in my workshops, and it would seem that this childhood loss is diminished only with difficulty.

The key factors influencing outcome appear to be personality in combination with the pre-existing relationship of dependence.

Social variables

Some loss alienates and isolates, while other loss produces gain. The gain may be freedom to leave a group or community or restrictions, for example those of a sexist relationship. If the person left was, or felt they were, an extension of the deceased and fed from their social network, the enormity of the loss becomes apparent.

Some religions and cultures will support the bereaved, showering them with offers of help and validation of their worth. In the UK there are diverse examples of community response to death; clear confrontation of it or avoidance may be apparent. How our social and cultural backgrounds influence our caring role will be explored in more detail later.

Whilst Christianity and other religions are usually assumed to be a help and support in sudden death, the bereaved may feel otherwise.

Miriam was 28 years of age when her 6-month-old baby died suddenly. She has one other child, aged $2^1/_2$ years, and is married to a solicitor. She is Jewish and has a large extended family living far and near. Her baby died quickly from overwhelming infection, at home in his cot. Miriam found him but was quickly removed from him.

Many people came and cried with her, and cared for her and her husband and the other child. Food and drink were brought and the housework done. Whatever she asked for she got. As is the custom, her baby boy was buried within 24 hours. Within a few days some of the activity had petered out but she described herself as being well cared for.

Years later Miriam feels as though something was not completed. She resents the 'indecent haste' that her religion inflicted upon her. She wanted to be with her dead baby and hold him, to have a chance to say goodbye. To actualize the loss in this way she feels would have helped her towards a more satisfactory coping state. She is resentful and angry that the rites of her religion prevented a more gentle separation that was somehow part of and under her control.

That day, events happened very quickly and she feels she was imposed upon, not only by the death but by the ritual that should have given her comfort in distress. It felt like intense activity that left her with nothing. She now feels that if there were a next time, she would have to choose between her apparent emotional needs and her religion.

Wordon (1991) emphasizes that intervention is best begun at the scene of the death. He describes help being offered 'aggressively'. It is no use saying 'how can I help you?'. Usually the bereaved do not know. A more assertive approach is to say 'I am here to talk to you and to work with you'.

In the past, much emphasis has been placed upon the importance of the opportunity to anticipate the death (Kubler-Ross 1969). Parkes (1975) also highlights this in his determinants of grief. However, we must not make the assumption that because someone has gone through a 'dying process' their death will not be perceived as sudden.

The role of anticipatory grief in helping people to cope with the grief process has been challenged. Fulton & Gottesman (1980) say that it has been confused conceptually with forewarning of loss. Anticipatory grief does not automatically occur after forewarning of loss. Fulton & Gottesman conclude that the usefulness of anticipatory grief is not determined by its duration, or by whether all the appropriate factors are present; it is the manner in which it is experienced and responded to by those concerned.

In looking at these determinants of grief, and at crisis intervention, I have identified two ways of providing a framework for working with sudden death. It is often difficult to establish a rapport with a client in crisis situations, because of the unusual and intense reactions we encounter — aspects of madness, chaos and disorder. The approaches described will, I believe, help to bring order where there is disorder, and restore meaning and insight where there seems to be madness. Some quality of life also needs to be restored. My search for other approaches is not over. Those discussed above highlight not only what may be useful, but also many difficulties. The immediate difficulties are explored in the next chapter.

Activity 1C

Make a plan of immediate actions which, after a sudden death, will help the client to:

1. have a realistic perception of the event
2. identify and access external resources
3. begin the process of finding inner resources.

REFERENCES

Bowlby J 1981 Loss, sadness and depression. Penguin, Harmondsworth
Caplan G 1964 Principles of preventive psychiatry. Basic Books, New York
Dubin W R, Sarnoff J R 1986 Sudden and unexpected death: interventions with survivors. Annals of Emergency Medicine 15(1):54–57
Erikson E H 1950 Childhood and society. W W Norton, New York
Fraser S, Atkins J 1990 Survivors' recollections of helpful and unhelpful emergency nurses' activities surrounding the sudden death of a loved one. Journal of Emergency Nursing 16(1):13–16
Fulton R, Gottesman D 1980 Anticipatory grief: a psychosocial concept reconsidered. British Journal of Psychiatry 137:45–54
Kubler-Ross E 1969 On death and dying. MacMillan, New York
Lindemann F 1944 Symptomatology and management of acute grief. American Journal of Psychiatry 101:141–149
Lundin T 1984 Long term outcome of bereavement. British Journal of Psychiatry 145:424–428
Murphy S A 1988 Mental distress and recovery in a high risk bereavement sample 3 years after untimely death. Nursing Research 37(1):30–35
Parkes C M 1975 Bereavement — studies of grief in adult life, 2nd edn. Penguin, Harmondsworth
Raphael B 1984 The anatomy of bereavement: a handbook for the caring professions. Hutchinson, London
Rogers M P, Reich P 1988 On the health consequences of bereavement. New England Journal of Medicine 319(8):510–511
Wordon J W 1991 Grief counselling and grief therapy, 2nd edn. Tavistock, London

2

The care on impact of death

As a counsellor of individuals and families at the immediate impact of a sudden death, I have noted that experiences at this time have a powerful effect on the whole process of grieving.

Many hours are later spent retracing the events of that fateful day. For those working only with the impact it is vital to know what help people value most at the time of the death, and how it influences the grieving process. In caring for people through the grieving process we need to know about the issues that stem from the impact.

The impact highlights areas of major vulnerability and of need that can help us provide care later in the grieving process. Difficulties encountered at the time of impact are often related to the responses of the helpers or the organization; these are dealt with in Chapters 6 and 8.

Much of this chapter is concerned with critical care units in hospitals, with an emphasis on Accident & Emergency departments, but the considerations discussed apply to any institutional setting. When people are away from familiar territory they experience a marked loss of autonomy and are in need of care and support.

The crisis begins with the arrival of the acutely ill or injured patient. If a relative or friend is not present, the hospital will have to contact someone, usually by telephone.

TELEPHONE NOTIFICATION

This will normally cause acute distress to the receiver of the information as well as to the worker. The dissociation of the receiver can lead him to fantasize and this is one of the worst circumstances in which to assimilate or process information.

Feelings of a person receiving information over the telephone frequently include the following:

'They knew more than they said'
'I am not sure what they said'
'It cannot be as bad as they say'
'I am not sure what they want me to do'
'It does not make sense'.

While fears of a worker giving information over the telephone include:

'I hope I have identified and am speaking to the right person'
'What if they collapse when I tell them, and they are alone?'
'Panic may prevent them from hearing me'
'What will I say if they ask me outright if their relative is dead?'
'People should not just hear this over the phone'
'We are less in control of the situation'.

Such a telephone call will be a crisis for many people. The situation will be unusual and upsetting and will disturb a person's steady state of equilibrium. It may be a new experience and they may not have the resources to deal with it. There will be difficulty in maintaining accurate cognitive perception (Caplan 1964).

It is therefore important to give crisis information under the best possible conditions for it to be received. One consideration is that the staff involved should share a concise set of defined terms (Robinson 1982). The basic terms for conveying the relative severity of situations are:

> critical   serious   fair   good

The meaning of these terms may not be common knowledge, but 'critical' will probably be understood.

If the patient has already died, most staff will want to convey this in person at the hospital so that the relative/friend can actualize the information by seeing the deceased. A dilemma will occur if the informer is asked over the phone if the patient has died, or is uncertain about whether to disclose over the phone that the patient has died. My experience is that if the hospital is quickly accessible it is better to tell people at the hospital. If they have a long distance to travel, and believe that by rushing they can be with their loved one before death or at the time of death, then it is essential to be honest over the phone.

Mrs James was telephoned at 11.00 pm by a hospital 200 miles from her home. She was told that her husband, who was working away, had been involved in a serious accident. Her first instinct was to ask how she could get to him, but she found herself asking tentatively, before the nurse could tell her, 'How is he?'. She then heard the worst: 'He is critically ill, having suffered multiple injuries'.

Mrs James told the nurse she would come as soon as she could. Her panic was compounded by the fact that her son was away on holiday. A neighbour and friend offered to drive her to the hospital, despite the unsocial hour. Even though she was able to drive she did not trust herself to do so alone.

Four hours later she arrived at the hospital after a fast and distressing drive through heavy rain. The worst was confirmed. She was too late, he had died. After another 2 hours of distress, and spending time with her deceased husband, she was ready to leave. She asked another nurse to confirm the time of her husband's death, and was angry to learn it was 20 minutes before the phone call.

Because of the cognitive disarray that this type of phone call produces, clear, concise information must be given:

- Say who you are, and from which hospital
- Be clear about who you are speaking to
- If this is not the most significant relative, where can he/she be found?
- Give the name of the ill or injured person, and their condition
- If there is doubt as to the identification, tell them you believe it is this person
- After telling them all this, check they are clear about
  - which hospital
  - how to get there
  - what you have said
- Then advise them
  - to get someone to come with them
  - to drive carefully and if necessary to get someone else to drive for them
  - to inform other close relatives or friends where they are heading.

Records of the time of the call, who responded and how, are important. After a death, some relatives will want to clarify the details.

Activity 2A

What would have been the advantages and disadvantages of informing Mrs James of her husband's death, in that first phone call from the hospital?

A ROOM FOR RELATIVES AND FRIENDS

Much of the feedback from relatives about their time in this room demonstrates how vulnerable they are. The word 'frightened' often comes into the conversation.

An advisory group for Bury Medical Audit (1994) told how relatives did not wish to be left alone unless they were assured that the nurse with them would be needed for the resuscitation. In the same document, many relatives felt the room to be claustrophobic, and they complained of its lack of windows. My own Accident & Emergency department's relatives' room has no outside wall, so a window on to the corridor has been installed. Relatives talked of feelings of isolation and how they preferred to witness some activity outside the room.

A joint working group of the British Association of A & E Medicine and the Royal College of Nursing (1994) emphasized the importance in this room of lighting, decoration and facilities. They recommend that in the room there should be:

- comfortable, domestic chairs and sofas. For people with special needs, for example the elderly, appropriate furniture should also be provided
- tissues
- ashtrays
- a telephone with direct dial access for incoming and outgoing calls
- telephone directories
- a wash basin, with soap, towel, mirror and freshen-up pack
- TV / radio available, but not prominent
- hot and cold drinks should be available; a fridge and kettle point enable independence, and are convenient for staff; a non-institutional tea/ coffee set should be provided
- toys and books for children.

Privacy as well as signs of activity and easy access to the patient were said to be important, as were curtains to prevent others outside witnessing distress. This combination may not be easy to achieve. It should also be remembered that a lot of people may arrive during an emergency and the room should accommodate up to ten people. Since they are often in a state of panic they need space, good light and ventilation.

THE VIGIL

An immediate need, whilst waiting or gaining access to the patient, is for information. The most frequent cause for complaint in one study was not being updated often enough after the initial information is given (Parrish et al 1987). This raises the question of who is best able to care for the relatives and to give them initial and updated information.

The person who cares for relatives within a hospital emergency department or other areas is usually a nurse, although some hospitals use a social worker or chaplain. Where crisis intervention is practised, or hospitals have liaison psychiatric departments, psychiatric nurses with special training in bereavement or crisis counselling may be involved. The nurse doing this work can also answer questions about the physical and emergency care, and the feelings associated with this.

It is difficult to separate discussion about the question of resuscitation and the imminent or possible loss from the feelings associated with it. For this reason I think a nurse is the best person for the immediate care, since she/he is likely to be able to liaise between the resuscitation room and the relatives more comfortably than most others. The nurse will also have some knowledge about the emergency treatment.

Relatives who were not present when the emergency occurred will need to identify the patient. This may involve finding a suitable moment during the resuscitation to take them to look at the patient in the resuscitation room. If the patient is going to the operating theatre quickly, it is important to establish positive identification first. This will mean that relatives do not have to sit with uncertainty for a long time. Even if you positively know the identity, relatives may not believe this until they have personally set eyes on the patient.

Any uncertainty will make things more difficult for the carer who will witness relatives expressing ideas that do not reflect the reality. Questions about injustice and guilt, and other profound and difficult issues, may arise:

'It cannot be him, we are so happy, everything is going so well for us now'
'Please tell me it is not true. He was due to be somewhere else at that time'
'I know it is him. It's not fair. Bad people live, why is this happening to
   us?'
'How can you believe in God when this happens?'
'Don't say any more. You are making a terrible mistake'.

Carers may experience great discomfort when confronted with issues they have previously avoided. It is difficult to be in the role of carer and supporter and yet not have the answers.

The nature of the injuries or illness may mean carers spending a prolonged period with the relatives before a patient dies or is pronounced dead. Serious head injuries, for example, may require brain scans, insertion of intracranial pressure measuring devices and neurosurgery. At some time during the process of care, the patient may die. News of procedures to be performed may give hope that is seized upon with unrealistic expectations. The patient going for insertion of a pacemaker may not survive and suddenly all hopes are dashed. This produces feelings that are very obviously conflicting.

Table 2.1 Survey of 100 sudden deaths — time spent by nurse with relatives of patient who subsequently died

Time spent	%
0–1 hour	27
1–2 hours	46
Over 2 hours	27
	100

The time spent with relatives whilst many resuscitation procedures were being carried out was measured for the 100 deaths in our study.

Table 2.1 shows that the time with the relatives on many occasions was 2 hours or more, which is a long time to witness and share another person's extremes of anguish and distress.

LOSS OF AUTONOMY

In these situations an overwhelming feeling of loss of autonomy is experienced by the relatives. The issue of advocacy for those in this vulnerable state is dealt with later. An awareness and sensitivity to the feelings of relatives and the way they are dealt with in the immediate term will have a significant effect on the process of grief in the long term.

It is necessary for most people to have some feeling of control over their lives. Plans, hopes and expectations give some feeling of comfort and movement. Suddenly, this is all thrown into chaos and confusion, pain and hurt:

Mrs Jones sat rigid in the relatives' room awaiting news of her son's condition. Paul was 8 years old, her only child. He had been hit by a bus when crossing the road on the way home from school. His friend had run home in panic to give the news of Paul's accident. A neighbour had confirmed that it was Paul, and an ambulance had taken him to the Accident & Emergency department.

The nurse told Mrs Jones that Paul's condition was critical, and asked if she wanted anyone to join her at the hospital. As her husband was away working, she asked for her mother and mother-in-law. Her words were almost inaudible. Now and again, she asked fearfully if there was any news.

When her mother and mother-in-law arrived, the nurse left for the resuscitation room to seek an update on Paul's condition. The team was talking of abandoning further efforts as there was no sign of life. The nurse was grateful that Paul did not look too bad as she returned to the relatives' room. Paul's mother looked so fragile and the nurse was frightened that further information would cause her to break. When she was told there was no improvement, and the outlook was poor, she just whispered 'Thank you'.

It was an hour after her arrival that a doctor joined Mrs Jones, the nurse and the family. Everyone knew the gravity of what he was going to say and yet hoped they would be wrong. 'Your son Paul has just died. I am very sorry.'

Paul's grandmothers wept openly and held Mrs Jones, distressed that their comfort evoked little or no response. The doctor carefully explained what measures had been taken to restore life and how it was to no avail. They thanked him for his efforts and Mrs Jones asked him flatly if Paul had suffered. She was confidently assured that he had not.

When the doctor left the room there was silence for a while and then Paul's mother asked, 'Can I see him?' The nurse's relief at this first reaction was mixed with anxiety at the distress Mrs Jones would feel. 'Yes, of course you can,' she said. Mrs Jones' mother quickly became very agitated: 'You must not do that. It is best to remember him as he was.' Her mother-in-law confirmed this: 'It won't do you any good — let's just go home.'

'I would like to see him,' Paul's mother whispered. The words did not convey the longing in her heart just to have another glimpse of his face. 'Just take it from me,' her mother said, 'You must not. You don't know about these things.' Her voice was desperate. She just wanted to get away. 'Why prolong the agony? We'll take her home,' they said to the nurse. The calm and sadness were rudely interrupted by Mrs Jones with a voice not previously heard. It was strong and determined: 'I want to see my little boy. Take me to him.' The nurse led her away.

When she returned to her mother and mother-in-law she was weeping and could not be consoled. Her cry was one of torment and questions. 'Why? Why?'

'We told you not to' they said.

When Mrs Jones was seen 10 months later she clearly remembered the struggle to see her son. She described how she nearly lost the battle, and how she had always believed in her mother's authority. Her struggle to speak, and wondering if she was being heard, was crystal clear to her. She had felt powerless and at the mercy of all around her, and her fate was to lose.

She does not know where she found the strength to state firmly what she wanted. The nurse had quickly used the opportunity to take her to see her son and, for this, she was very grateful. She wanted to be with him and quickly, and was glad she could see him just where he was when he died. Her memory is of him lying on the resuscitation table draped in a white sheet, and seeing the shape of his genitals under the sheet. When she saw this and his washed, white face she knew it was her little boy. She held his hand, wept and said goodbye to him.

Now, 10 months later, she clearly knows the value of this time and how she was nearly denied it. The loss is borne alone, however, as Paul's death is a taboo subject with her husband. Her comfort comes from her remembered joys with Paul and her goodbye. The value of the goodbye is simple to her; since her childhood she has believed that anyone injured in this way would be squashed flat. To carry this image around with her would have been torment and misery. She knows, as I do, that for most people, reality is far more acceptable than fantasy. Fantasies are bizarre and cruel, and can be uncontrollable. Reality gave her comfort. Reality confronted her with the starkness of death, but it was still preferable to her long-held belief of flattened people.

This period of waiting and separation reinforces loss of autonomy, and most people describe the time as being very distressing. The notion of helplessness, being immobilized or stuck and unable to make choices, underlies most of the problems for which individuals seek help. There is evidence that belief in increased personal control will have long-term benefits (Furlong 1981). Helpers need to examine ways of giving clients some control or choice.

ACCESS DURING RESUSCITATION

Relatives may have been present when the accident occurred or the illness became life threatening and, at the scene or in the ambulance, will have witnessed their loved one being actively resuscitated. It may be difficult to separate them from the patient as the patient enters the resuscitation area.

Distress is increased by separation from their loved one (Renner 1991). The main issue for them, particularly if the patient dies, is that they failed the patient by not being there at their death. Many doctors believe there is no reason why relatives should not watch resuscitation (Adams et al 1994). It should be noted that medical staff able to cope with this are usually senior, well-experienced doctors. Others suggest that it produces too much anxiety for junior doctors, and that often an invasive procedure is involved which would cause unreasonable distress for the relatives (Schilling 1994).

A study from the Foote Hospital surveyed 47 family members present during a resuscitation (Hanson & Strawser 1992). Of these, 76% felt that their adjustment to the death was made easier by their presence in the room. Thirty respondents (64%) felt their presence was beneficial to the dying person. Many were sure the dying person had heard them express their love and goodbyes. This is most important as far as healing the grief is concerned (Parkes 1975). Another study (Doyle et al 1987) concluded that there appears to be no reason for continuing policies which exclude family members. This paper talks about it being an option, which indicates giving relatives a choice.

It should be emphasized that the presence of relatives may produce distress for medical staff (Zoltie et al 1994). Chalk (1995) suggests that all staff should be in agreement on this issue, and discusses the importance of someone being able to inform and care for the relatives exclusively. In addition, staff need to care for each other. Dealing with the relatives' loss of autonomy, and being aware of the value of doing so, needs to be balanced by recognition of staff needs and efforts to make it more manageable for them.

BREAKING BAD NEWS

If relatives are not present when the patient dies, or if they arrive after the death, staff will have to break the news to them. The first contact doctors have with the relatives in most cases is to break the bad news. It is felt that final confirmation of death must come from the doctor's own mouth, although there are occasions when it is the nurse who does this. For the doctor, it is usually a transaction with strangers at a critical time in the strangers' lives. The nurse will, by this stage, have established some rapport with the relatives and should always be present when they are given the news.

In our study we asked relatives how they felt about the way the news was given. Many of the relatives felt the doctors performed very badly when they spent the usual brief time with the relatives. The doctor may have taken a long time to give them the awful news. Some doctors ask various questions about the patient's past medical history and then give the news. Others go into a preamble prior to the final words. Relatives have expressed anger at such treatment.

The main criticism we encountered was of communication skills. One woman described the doctor as: 'Performing like a bus conductor, swaying on both legs with one hand on the door post and looking into the distance.' Table 2.2 shows the results of a survey into the length of time doctors spent with relatives after breaking the bad news. Most negative remarks were about the doctor not sitting down and being on the same level when the news was delivered. Many people commented on poor eye contact. Some relatives continued to complain about how the news was given, and had difficulty accepting the reality of the loss.

The use of euphemisms for death is to be avoided. Words such as dead or died are unequivocal. The often-used phrases:

Table 2.2 Survey of 100 sudden deaths — time spent by doctors with relatives, after giving confirmation of death

Time spent	%
0–5 minutes	51
6–15 minutes	23
15 minutes or over	8
Doctor not used at all	18
	100

- He has passed on
- He has slipped away
- We have lost her

may be well meaning but are open to misinterpretation or may feed someone's denial. One man told us:

When the doctor came in and said I am afraid we have lost her, I thought what a damned fool. How could they allow a woman who is so sick to leave the hospital? You see, my wife was always a bit wayward and if someone said something she did not want to hear she would just walk out.

I remember saying, "What do you mean? How could you just let her walk out?" He looked embarrassed, and said she is dead. I remember being angry and saying: "Well, why didn't you say so?"

A study of the parents of critically ill children admitted to hospital (Farrell & Frost 1992) found that, although the information they received was distressing and traumatic, there was an overwhelming need to know that it was correct and honest.

Frequently the person communicating the bad news feels they have done it badly. Communication is a dynamic, complex, continuous exchange. In stressful circumstances, it is difficult for the message to be perceived and assimilated. Powerful feelings interfere with the process. To complicate matters further, the encounter is often between strangers. We all fear the unknown. Whilst some responses are expected, a wide range of human feelings can emerge under stress. Strong feelings of ineffectiveness, and being at a loss as to which direction to follow, are experienced.

A training package for junior doctors (British Medical Association 1992) showed how the doctor breaking the bad news can feel he or she made a complete mess of it. The package goes on to stress that training, mentorship and support are essential. Initially, the recipient of the news may experience shock, disbelief and an inability to accept the loss. These are all part of the normal grieving process. At the time the bad news is given, all these feelings may be experienced at once. Lindemann (1944) described how acute grief was compounded by waves of somatic distress lasting 20–60 minutes, for example decreased muscular power, a feeling of emptiness in the stomach, tightness of the throat, choking, shortness of breath, sighing, perspiring, flushed face and finally exhaustion or fainting. The bearer of the bad news may feel that by saying what they did they have inflicted this intense pain on the recipient.

Activity 2B

Make a list of the words which are used instead of 'died' or 'dead'. Mark those you might use, and explore how these are open to misinterpretation.

Whilst the loss is the real focus of the event, there is a definite need for clear, understandable information. In a situation which is outside the realms of understanding, there is a strong need to introduce some sense of order and to remove some of the perplexity.

Honest, direct information about the sequence of events, from people who do not skirt around the real issues is valued by clients. It is an important factor in encouraging a realistic perception of the crisis event. However, this information involves some confrontation. The recipient may show a degree of cognitive disarray as a result. This leads us on to the second component of the management of crisis — external resources.

HELP TO FIND IMMEDIATE RESOURCES

Some extremely simple tasks become very difficult or complicated at times of crisis. Information habitually familiar to people can become difficult to locate. Family, friends or significant others, though geographically near, may seem far away. Those who are far away will cause the helplessness and frustration to intensify.

For example, people familiar with telephone directories will ask you to find someone's number, because they cannot understand its sequence. It is not at all uncommon for people not to be able to use the telephone or dial a number. Which persons are significant in their lives, and how you can arrange for them to join you, is an important issue. It often requires painstaking discussion to elicit where these people are.

It is important in a large and busy Emergency department that relatives and friends are able to ask for a named member of staff on arrival. To arrive distressed and find that reception staff do not know who you are puts both staff and relatives in a difficult position. It also suggests that this most significant of events is not given priority.

Some relatives will negotiate with the carer prior to the arrival of others as to who should give them the bad news. I feel it is important that they impart this information to the new arrivals. Carers must encourage this, reluctant though they may be.

ARRIVAL OF THE RELATIVES

The arrival of other relatives and friends will produce some intense distress and a feeling for the carer of beginning it all again. The events leading to the death and why it happened will be reviewed, perhaps more than once. The carer may use this opportunity to evaluate how the person who was at the hospital from the start perceives and relates to the event. Allowing people to relate events to those who join them, will again confront them and give them an opportunity to review the death.

When the story is repeated other things may well be clarified. Other family and friends arriving may give further opportunity to spend time with the deceased. This is often a time when all the pain and anguish becomes apparent. The family may need to be together alone, but do not assume they want to, check first.

ADVOCACY

The most significant person in the deceased's life may now be at risk from being swamped with care. People often recall the problem this caused them, as will be discussed later. If a person has been alone with the immediate grief, it is as if this must be compensated for and the people arriving must take over responsibility for them. They begin to answer for them, they make decisions for them, they direct them in any way possible.

One of the roles of the carer in this immediate situation is to protect the bereaved from this, and it will be resisted by the additional people if all that they can give in the situation is to be seen to be in control. It will be more of an issue where the arriving relative is a male caring for a female. In a life crisis such as this the immediate pain and chaos seem unbearable. Attempts to replace it with some order and control may involve a loss of autonomy for the person closest to the deceased.

You may now be beginning to appreciate how time consuming or complex the care provision can seem when families are large and when many other people arrive on the scene. If this suggests it is all too difficult to undertake, we need to return to the question why do it? The message that is most important and should be uppermost in our minds about this immediate care is as follows. The bereaved person will never again have the chance to work through this most difficult time; they must be given the space and time to in the immediate term. It is an opportunity to begin the normal process of grieving and should not be lost.

The advocacy role of the carer is an important one. Advocacy provides individuals with the help and support they need to pursue their own interests. It will help them to find a voice when they have difficulty speaking for themselves. It will often deal with a conflict of interests such as relatives overriding the needs of the bereaved.

Relatives or friends will often take a carer aside or clearly have a need to speak to them alone. They are at a loss as to how they will care for or cope with the distress of the bereaved, and they will often want direction on this. Some questions are about definite issues: 'Should I take her home

Activity 2C

Why may the needs of one family member conflict with those of another in this situation?

with me?' Others are more difficult with no clear answer: 'What can I say to her about this?'

The distress or helplessness of the friend or relative often leaves a carer feeling as anxious for them as for the bereaved. One should be prepared to give relatives some time and opportunity to talk about their anxiety if this is possible. The task is now becoming even more difficult. Needs of individuals are increasingly diverse and confrontation situations can easily arise.

ABSENT AT THE TIME OF DEATH

Because most sudden deaths require vigorous attempts to resuscitate the patient, relatives are not often present at the time of death. Many will not be present in the hospital, and others will be kept waiting in a different room. The majority will ask, when death is confirmed:

'Did he suffer?'
'Did he know what was happening?'
'Did he say anything?'

Some people can place the focus more precisely on the issue most important to them and say:

'Did he ask or say anything about me?'

Strong ambivalence is expressed at not being present at the time of death — a great need to have been there and an equally great need to run in the opposite direction. When this ambivalence has settled, many will regret or feel guilt at not having been present.

Carers can give clear information and should not avoid answering questions. Often they will be confirming that the patient was unconscious and had no awareness of what was happening around him. At other times they will be informing them that strong analgesic drugs were given to deal with the pain. Supplementary information about the nature of these drugs is helpful, and can alleviate further distress. We may also say: 'The drug was a powerful narcotic, like morphine.' Most people have heard of morphine and understand its useful properties.

Despite all these reassurances, issues such as why they did not get to the person on time, and their helplessness in trying to facilitate this, can become prolonged difficulties for the people who are left. Because of the value for most people of being present at the time of death, we must not forget waiting relatives when attempts at resuscitation have failed. Some patients will continue to have a heartbeat for a short time after attempts have ceased. The relatives can be brought to the patient to spend a short time with them before they die.

The separation of family from patient has been identified as causing difficult and often disruptive aggression in emergency departments (Wright 1993). Work in a USA hospital explored whether relatives should be present whilst resuscitation was taking place (Doyle et al 1987). It was found that relatives may wish to be with family members who may be dying, even though resuscitation efforts are being made. Seventy people who participated in the study were taken to the resuscitation room, accompanied by a member of staff, who explained what was happening. None of the participants interfered with the resuscitation efforts.

The participants were later contacted, and 47 responded. Of those respondents who had been present during the resuscitation, 44 (94%) felt they would want to participate again. The study found that relatives present during resuscitation felt that they had been able to help the person undergoing resuscitation. This in turn was helpful in the grieving process. The authors saw no reason for continuation of policies that exclude family members from the resuscitation room.

When resuscitation efforts are discontinued and there is still a heartbeat it is important to disconnect the patient from the monitor, otherwise relatives watch the monitor and it can cause problems of concentration in the interaction with the patient. Witnessing the trace 'going flat', can cause alarm and distress. It is also best to remove intubation tubes and intravenous lines. If it is not possible for relatives to be present at time of death, most appreciate seeing the deceased as soon as possible afterwards.

SEDATION

Requests for sedation when suffering the acute distress of grief after a sudden death seem to be becoming less common than say 10 years ago. Some people will check it out by asking: 'Is it still thought to be harmful to sedate someone in this situation?'

The most grief-stricken person, in the immediate throes of a sudden death, rarely asks for sedation for themselves. It is usually requested by someone close to them, and if this person overhears he usually rejects the idea vehemently. The request for sedation may really be an attempt to relieve the distress of the accompanying person on witnessing pain.

Most people who have been sedated or taken tranquillizers will recount the problems this has caused them. Many of those I have seen for bereavement counselling have regretted the recourse to drugs for coping with their grief. It is to be avoided if at all possible.

I firmly believe that the truth sets people free of some of the pain. For the nurses, taking people to touch, talk to and sit with the deceased is painful and time-consuming. Confirmation of its value is therefore important. Clients often speak of the value and ambivalent feelings of spending time with the deceased. Not one person in our study expressed negative feelings about spending time with the dead person. Many had regrets at not doing so and for some the thoughts they conjured up about how the unseen deceased looked were cruel and tormenting.

Relatives in this situation do need someone to act as advocate for them. This will be useful in the long term but they will rarely ask for it. They are uncertain of what is allowed and what the rules of the organization are. They might have lived with someone for 20 years but are unsure if they can ask to be with them and for how long. Another thought they have is that we have too much to do for the living without spending too long on the dead.

One elderly lady said: 'I was so grateful when the nurse said there may be things you want to say to your husband. I did not know, you see, if you were allowed to or if they would think I was barmy talking to someone dead. It made it natural, it made it all right. She held his hand when we went in to him and she said I could. You do not know what you can do, what is allowed. It was very special for me having that time together. He was my husband after all, but we need to be told what we can do.'

Once through the doors of an institution the patient is no longer entirely the family's or the individual's concern. They relinquish part of him to the organization, are reluctant to state their own needs and do not know what boundaries are imposed upon their needs and behaviour. The carers are needed to facilitate and encourage normal requests. An insight into the constraints that people perceive is necessary, but it is not enough. We have to state clearly what is possible in explicit terms:

'You can hold his hand if you want to.'
'Feel free to talk if you have things to say.'
'I am sure you want to say goodbye.'

Individual autonomy may also be compromised over the issue of viewing the body. One of my greatest challenges has been helping young widows to realize their immediate needs. Young wives often, and quite naturally, have a need to hold and weep and share last moments with husbands. However, it is not uncommon for older male relatives or male friends of the husband, to tell them they must go home and it would be better if they did not do it. This profoundly disadvantaged person, rendered weak and ineffective with no control over her life, usually accedes to the other's apparent strength and knowledge.

Perhaps men do this because they need to be seen to be taking control. Will the distress produced by a wife's contact with the body be too difficult to control or witness? I believe that these men's underlying need is to look after themselves or to be seen to take positive action in a very difficult situation. Once they have taken this stance it is difficult to convince them otherwise. To invite contact with the dead person appears to be imposing pain and distress on someone already very distressed. The easy way out is to let someone take over.

The ritual of a short vigil and goodbyes is a healthy and positive start to leaving someone behind. The bereaved need our help to begin this journey. The prevention of contact with the deceased creates problems for mothers who have experienced sudden infant death syndrome or other infant and child deaths. This overprotection, though well meaning, can have long-lasting implications. It must be re-emphasized that not one person in our study had regrets at seeing and spending time with the deceased. Being aware of this, we can help the bereaved to verbalize and focus on needs that are difficult for them to assert.

Discouraging time with the body may be linked to staff avoiding this painful area and also to the resources and time it demands. Opposition to a vigil from mortuary staff, and struggles with relatives of the bereaved do occur. This difficulty in confrontation with the reality of the death may be a characteristic of Western culture. Whatever the underlying cause, we must take into account the feedback we have from bereaved people regarding immediate needs.

IDENTIFICATION

For legal reasons, many sudden death victims need formal identification in the presence of a police officer. This is always so for cot deaths and other trauma victims. It may be performed when relatives go to sit with the deceased and the police officer discreetly withdraws after the initial contact. The officer will later obtain a statement to the effect that they identified the deceased in his presence. If this identification is neglected, the relatives will have to return to the hospital or mortuary and repeat the viewing. This needs explaining to relatives. Many prefer to separate the more formal procedure from their own time with the deceased and from their goodbyes.

PROPERTY

One woman, when visited 10 months later, asked the researcher to help her remove from the bottom of the wardrobe a bag of clothes given to her on the day of the death. This request appeared symbolic of the stage this lady had reached in her grieving process.

Some relatives complained that they were not asked to take away clothing, and others said they were, despite the fact that it may have been cut or bloodstained. It became apparent that some nurses felt the family should be given the opportunity to take away the clothing, whilst other families were protected from this. Although presentable white cardboard carrier bags were available, many people were given the clothes in a white plastic bag. This took on a great significance:

'I went in with a wife and came out with a dustbin liner of clothes.'

'They just stuffed his clothes into a dustbin bag without folding them properly.'

People attached hidden meanings to this, and some felt it reflected the sort of care received. It is an example of how an issue, distant from the main focus, can take on enormous significance.

To arrive at the hospital with a person and to leave, after the death, with a few possessions, confronts the bereaved with the reality of that person having been left behind. For this reason, I prefer it to be part of the immediate care and not postponed until later. Nurses often insist that they do explain when clothing has been cut from the patient to gain access for resuscitation, perhaps they do not always make this clear because it deals with a difficult or distasteful aspect of the death.

DOCUMENTS

Along with this handing over the property, relatives are given a booklet about what to do after a death (DSS). We also give a list of information produced by the hospital on how to register the death and obtain a death certificate. This shifts the focus to practical aspects of the loss and often produces a marked change in emotional response. There is a sense of control and the need to 'get on with the practical details.'

Responses at this stage often refer to practicalities: 'I will have to carry on somehow.' Another response is to depersonalize the loss. This may be expressed as: 'Of course this is a common occurrence for you' or 'People die every day and others have to get on with it.' The emphasis has moved to a national or global problem. Another common response is to turn the attention to the nurse:

'How do you cope with doing this all the time?'
'What an awful job you have.'
'This is just part of the job, is it?'

The shift from the personal meaning of a death, and the need to put it into some other perspective, may prove difficult for the carer. It may be welcomed as a move away from the personal pain, but can mean entering into difficult areas such as the meaning of sudden death. The idea that this little scenario is being played out all over the world in many varying locations, is frequently reflected upon. The carer may be questioned on the meaning of death and feel uncomfortable at not having the answers to questions such as:

'How do others cope with this?'
'Why now?'
'Is there some message for me somewhere in all of this?'

At this stage the family may request the services of a chaplain or other religious support, or it may be offered to them. In sudden death, it is not unusual for the response to be anger, and you must be prepared for this. It is important that the likelihood of such a response does not prevent you making the offer. It is important that people are given the opportunity to express this emotion.

LEAVING THE HOSPITAL OR PLACE OF DEATH

Prior to their leaving, carers may want to check that the relatives have all property or items of jewellery that were with the deceased. It will be a time to confirm they know what procedures to follow next. It is important to check that they know who to contact to clarify what may have happened or for more information.

No one should be allowed to leave alone if at all possible. In the past 12 years I have only known one man insist on this. Help in arranging transport, or obtaining a taxi, should be given. Leaving presents great difficulty for most people; once the initial feeling of wanting to take flight has diminished, people often feel the opposite. It is hard to leave their loved one behind. This is often expressed in a comment such as: 'Take care of him, please.'

The final act, in dealing with the immediate needs of the relatives, is helping them to leave. We can acknowledge their difficulty: 'I know it is hard for you to leave him here.' They will be confronted with the separation and loss in this part of the procedure. It is often the trigger for a re-emergence of overt distress. It is an opportunity for the carer to say how sorry they are that they could not do more to help them. It may be the final confirmation of awareness and distress at the awful outcome for them. People appear to value this being acknowledged.

The process of immediate care is time consuming and emotionally very demanding on the carer. How we pick up the pieces, both for ourselves and the organization, is discussed later.

To reiterate, this chapter has looked at apparent and implicit component parts of the immediate care of relatives where there has been a sudden death. Because in the immediate term the grief-stricken person is put at a disadvantage, because he does not know what to ask for, because he has been left weak, impotent and sometimes speechless, we must meet unspoken needs.

Activity 2D

- Make a list of your goals of care at the impact of the death.
- Who is 'responsible' if the goals are not achieved?

REFERENCES

Adams S, Whitlock M, Higgs R, Bloomfield P, Baskett P J F 1994 Should relatives be allowed to watch resuscitation? British Medical Journal 308:1687–1689
British Association of A & E Medicine and Royal College of Nursing 1994 Bereavement care in A & E departments. RCN, London
British Medical Association 1992 A stressful shift. BMA Board of Science and Education, London
Bury Medical Audit 1994 Audit of the care of bereaved relatives following sudden death. 121 Silver Street, Bury BL9 OEN, UK
Caplan G 1964 Principles of preventive psychology. Basic Books, New York
Chalk A 1995 Should relatives be present in the resuscitation room? Journal of A & E Nursing 3(2):58–61
Doyle C, Post H, Burney R E, Maino J, Keefe M, Rhee K J 1987 Family participation during resuscitation — an option. Annals of Emergency Medicine 16(6):673–675
Farrell M F, Frost C 1992 The most important needs of parents of critically ill children: parents' perception. Journal of Intensive Care and Critical Care Nursing 8(3):130–139
Furlong F W 1981 Determinism and free will: a review of the literature. American Journal of Psychiatry 138:435
Hanson C, Strawser D 1992 Family presence during cardio-pulmonary resuscitation: Foote Hospital's 9-year perspective. Journal of Emergency Nursing 18(2): 104–106
Lindemann E 1944 Symptomatology and management of acute grief. American Journal of Psychiatry 101(2):141–148
Parkes C M 1975 Determinants of outcome following bereavement. Omega Journal of Death & Dying 6(4):303–323
Parrish G A, Holden K S, Skiendzielewski J J 1987 Emergency department experience with sudden death: a survey of survivors. Annals of Emergency Medicine 16:792–796
Renner S 1991 I desperately needed to see my son. British Medical Journal 302:356
Robinson M A 1982 Telephone notification of emergency and critical care patients. Annals of Emergency Medicine 11:616–618
Schilling R J 1994 Should relatives watch resuscitation? British Medical Journal 309:406
Whitlock M, Baskett P, Bloomfield P, Higgs R, Adams S 1994 Should relatives be allowed to watch resuscitation? British Medical Journal 308:1687–1692
Wright B 1993 Caring in crisis 2nd edn. Churchill Livingstone, Edinburgh
Zoltie N, Sloan J, Wright B 1994 Observed resuscitation may affect a doctor's performance. British Medical Journal 309:406

Everybody has a story to tell

In many cases in psychiatry the patient who comes to us has a story that is not told, and which as a result, no one knows of. To my mind therapy only really begins after the investigation of that wholly personal story. It is the patient's secret, the rock against which he is shattered. If I know his secret story, I have a key to the treatment.

Carl Jung 1961 Memories, dreams, reflections.
Vintage, New York

The process of reliving the events of the day of the death is an essential part of the grief process. Later in this chapter I describe how the people in our study told their story of the day their loved one died suddenly. First I would like to explore story-telling and its therapeutic value.

STORY-TELLING

Communication is an important aspect of human behaviour. It is also important in implementing the process of caring. One of our major roles is to help clients through telling their stories, to explore the circumstances of their lives to resolve the things that have gone wrong.

In social situations we tell our stories with some superficiality. In a therapeutic relationship we may develop a facilitative intimacy which differs from social intimacy. Socially, people tell stories to one another. In facilitative relationships only the client is involved in the story-telling. Clients not only tell the story of the events in their lives and the circumstances these events produce, but do so with a purpose in mind. The change to a therapeutic intimacy can be difficult initially, since it violates social taboos. It is a move from social chitchat into areas of serious concern for the client.

The literature of folklore, myth and fairy tales contains a multitude of stories that client groups can use for insight (Huelskoetter & Murray 1991). The stories can help clients to explore their own lives.

As the feedback from our study showed, the worker available on the day of the death has a very important role. The client is not constrained by social intimacy with the worker, and quickly values the facilitative intimacy. The bereaved person is often entangled with family dynamics and social constraints, and values an objective viewpoint. I am always amazed at the degree of disclosure achieved, and the way this leads to an intimacy not usually established so quickly. For example, within 10 minutes a complete stranger revealed to me:

'How will I live without him? I loved him so much. He was everything to me. It is not fair leaving me like this just when everything was going so well. How could he do it? I hate him for it.'

Within a short period of time powerful intimate details are disclosed which, when later reviewed by the client, surprise them. When they re-tell their story the worker is an integral part of the intimacies of the event. Some staff find this makes them uncomfortable and they feel they are intruding into people's personal lives. They could not imagine themselves disclosing intimacies to a stranger after such a short period of time. Make no mistake about it, the worker becomes a key person in the story.

Picard (1990) acknowledges the compelling nature of what must be told, and how this helps to heal the pain. She describes the story as a narrative of events which is on-going. After the disaster at Lockerbie, amidst a flurry of activity and confusion, the professional carers asked themselves 'what will we do when we get to the people involved?' (McKechnie 1993). They arrived at one simple answer: 'Just let them tell their story'.

McKechnie relates that no pre-existing script is being performed; on the contrary, the stories unfold. They are discovered in the process of telling, and are told slowly. It is important to facilitate this process. Some of the principles and practices involved in facilitating intimacy are discussed next.

RESPONDING TO THE CLIENT'S STORY

Five aspects of responding can be identified as follows:

Responding with empathy. This is the ability to feel the feelings of other people so that one can respond to and understand their experiences on their terms. Empathy is distinguished from sympathy by lack of agreement or pity or condolence. Without empathy there is no real basis for helping.

Responding with respect. This indicates we value the integrity of the client and have faith in them to solve their problems, given appropriate help. We have respect for their ability to take charge of their own destiny.

Being genuine in response. This is the ability to be real or honest with one another, but I do not suggest that honesty is always the best policy if it is brutal or if the client is not ready to deal with it. Genuine response is based on a relationship we have had time to evaluate and develop. If we are real, our clients can risk being real themselves. Being genuine involves risk and is not always being safe and socially acceptable. Hopefully the client will mirror this.

Responding with warmth. This is closely linked with empathy and respect. Warmth and intimacy cannot be forced, and can be difficult for some clients to handle, especially if they have had little of this in their lives. We accept the client's right to distance, and convey warmth mostly by respect and empathy.

Responding with immediacy. This is responding to what is here and now. We begin with what the client is experiencing in starting or developing the therapeutic relationship. This acknowledges the immediate difficulties.

It is the province of knowledge to speak and it is the privilege of wisdom to listen.

Oliver Wendell Holmes
The poet at the breakfast table 1872 Ch 10

LISTENING TO THE CLIENT'S STORY

Listening is often underrated. It requires skill, patience, understanding and perseverance.

Listening and hearing should be distinguished. A voluntary effort to understand what is being said requires listening. Hearing is the audible reception of the spoken word. People need to know not only that we are listening but that we have heard. This suggests that listening is active rather than passive. We must convey a desire to hear what the client is saying.

The client knows we hear him from our verbal and non-verbal indications, for example, leaning forward, good eye contact (not staring), nods,

Activity 3A
Think of a recent encounter with someone and describe: 1. what helped you listen 2. what prevented you from listening.

frowns and smiles. Our questions or responses will indicate to the client whether we have been listening to them.

We may need a clear, standardized history of the event. But this could discourage the client from spontaneously expressing himself. On the other hand an overpermissiveness with little feedback from the listener may mean that the interaction lacks direction and cohesion. Remember that this story telling also has therapeutic goals.

A response from the listener which is too passive can convey a lack of interest or competence. Some inappropriate messages are conveyed to the client when responses are wrongly timed. If we make a quick assumption about the knowledge and verbal skills of the client, our feedback or questions may confuse them. We should not assume the client knows more or less than he actually does.

Messages that lack clarity, simplicity and directness are inefficient. They will confuse or complicate the process and use up valuable energy. Crisis stories drain the teller of energy. Pace will be important: we must not demand too much too soon.

The listener may experience errors of perception, missing vital clues. We must be careful not to respond only to content and thereby miss messages of effect. Our own psychological or physical discomfort may make us inattentive. We can misinterpret the meaning of the message. This is usually due to lack of information or because we view it in terms of our own value system. Rather than being open to the speaker, we are judging them on the basis of our personal experience or beliefs.

Errors in feedback often stem from problems in listening. This kind of listening may be simple but because it has therapeutic goals it is important not to misinterpret what you learn. Being open and honest with the client about our difficulties of perception will normally be appreciated:

'I am not sure I understand that'
'Am I right in thinking that ..?'

COMMUNICATION SKILLS

My own experience of listening to these stories is that in the first or second telling of the story I have been less active in my responses. As the number of sessions progresses I have used more facilitative communication skills. Let us consider these next:

Reflecting content. In reflecting the content of part of the story, the listener gives the client the opportunity to hear what they have said. This can, however, be overused.

Reflecting feeling. 'It sounds like you felt really angry or abused by this'. This attempts to identify meanings that clarify or distort difficulties. The client is often encouraged to make additional comments that enlighten further — 'Yes, I never realized how strongly I felt about that'.

Giving information. It is common for the client to ask 'What do you think?', 'What should I have done?'. It is not always useful to answer them with another question. Some information is straightforward: 'The agency to help with that is ...'. Or it could be 'I have known other people, in similar situations, do the same'. Some clients need help to normalize their feeling or behaviour.

Clarifying. This is an attempt to understand the client's statement. 'I am not sure what you mean'. Illustrations are useful qualifiers.

Paraphrasing. Assimilating and re-stating what the client has said. 'I hear you saying you cannot stand people remarking how well you are coping'. This is a chance to test our understanding of what the client is trying to say.

Questioning. A more direct way of speaking to the client. When used excessively it is controlling; it can also narrow down the nature and range of responses. Questions can be open-ended to allow freedom of response, or closed to allow only 'yes' or 'no'.

Summarizing. This can be done during a session but is usually helpful at the end to assess how the time was used. Some listeners to stories use it to start a session if the client has difficulty beginning. A short summary with the question 'Is that how you see it?' can help them make a start.

In 1994 I received the following letter, which I have the writer's permission to publish:

Dear Mr Wright

In September 1980 my husband, affectionately known as Curly, died when the ship he was working on, the mv *Derbyshire*, sank off the coast of Japan. At the time there were no counselling services available. Unfortunately there was no one available to talk to me who had any experience of my type of bereavement. My husband had died overseas, there was no body and no funeral.

I decided that one day, I would tell someone how I managed to cope and survive. That day has now arrived. For most of the time I have had no one to talk to. Living so far from the sea, local people do not fully understand my problem. Comments such as 'Well, you were used to him being away, you're used to being on your own' quickly confirmed this. Consequently I kept a diary and from this I have extracted my personal story. I have omitted details of the problems experienced by my three children.

Last June an expedition found the ship, lying nearly 3 miles down. This was confirmed when video pictures shown by Channel Four News clearly found part of the name of the ship '...SHIRE'. In August I made a private visit to Okinawa to say my goodbyes to Curly. It was a wonderful experience and it has changed me completely. Friends have even said I look and sound different! When I returned home, a friend whose father was on the *Derbyshire* rang and asked if I thought it would help her to go to Japan. She also explained that she was unable to talk about her father and her feelings regarding his death. I compiled this booklet to show her I hadn't just made the decision, written a cheque and flown to Okinawa. A great deal of hard work had gone into my decision, hence the title of my booklet 'My long road to Japan'.

My decision to send a copy to you was influenced by my attendance at one of your seminars in Cambridge. Perhaps you would be kind enough to let me know if my story makes sense to you, as someone who does not know me or my story. Please keep this copy and use it to further your knowledge and experience. I would be grateful to know if and how you are able to use it. If I am able to help you in any way, please don't hesitate to get in touch with me. If my experiences can be of assistance to others similarly affected, or to those suffering a bereavement where there is no body, then I would be willing to help.

Yours sincerely
Marion Bayliss

Near the beginning of her story, Marion states:

It's a confusing time. So many things float around my brain, but are not yet ready to emerge. I think I know why water on television, rough sea, sounds, etc. trouble me. Cannot put feelings into words yet. It confuses me, though I will overcome it during 1993 (hopefully). The difficulty lies in not really knowing how to start, especially regarding the water. Actually it's a big step in recognizing the needs.

Her written story ends:

I feel I have a more relaxed relationship with Curly now, which seems more healthy. I can never forget him but now I am able to look to the future. I feel that now, I am able to hold fast to these sure things, the love of family, and that I can really enjoy and be aware of that dawn that lights a new day.

Marion's is a powerful, unique story. She demonstrates well how the story unfolded and clarified events, and how she became liberated when she was able to tell her story.

REVIEWING THE EVENTS OF 'THAT DAY'

When the relatives in our study were visited later, they were asked to describe the care given to them in the immediate situation. This care had some link with the grieving process, as can be seen in what the relatives

Activity 3B
What prevents us from having a realistic perception of an event?

Table 3.1   Causes of death in our 100 sudden deaths

Cause	No.
Medical, i.e. cardiac arrest, subarachnoid haemorrhage, etc.	63
Road traffic accident	12
*Suicide	7
Sports	2
Work accident	4
Home accident	3
Surgical emergency	1
Cot death	8

*This was atypical

told us. The process of reliving that day, and describing the events, also had some interesting repercussions. Some of the insights gained by people, and by ourselves in retrospect, are described next. Certain kinds of sudden death were identified as resulting in more pain and long-term difficulties (see Table 3.1 for a list of the causes of death in our study).

We wrote to 100 people recorded as next-of-kin where there had been a sudden death. The typed letter was short and to the point, and a stamped addressed envelope was enclosed. The letter was signed by me and came from the department where the death had been confirmed, i.e. the Accident & Emergency Department. The letter simply asked if we could visit them to discuss what happened to them at the hospital on the day their loved one had died. We stated that the purpose was to try to improve the care we gave to relatives when a sudden death had occurred. A consent form was included with the letter, and we requested an address or telephone number at which they could be contacted. Permission was given to use the information for the purpose of the study.

Although the case studies in this book are based on fact, names and details have been altered to protect the identity of the people involved. Only one person expressed any anxiety about confidentiality and how the material would be used. People were very keen that it be used to help others in a similar situation. The response rate was high despite the sensitive nature of the material (Table 3.2). One of the conditional responses was 'Only if you do not bring medical students.'

Table 3.2   Survey of 100 sudden deaths — responses on being asked to discuss the sudden death

Response	%
Signed response to agree to be seen	51
Letters returned by Post Office 'Gone Away'	4
Conditional response, e.g.	4
'Only without my husband'	
'Only with my husband'	
Objection or angry response	1
No response	40

An interesting point is that the returns showed that a number of people had moved house. This change of house is an issue often discussed in my bereavement counselling. Is it best to move quickly or wait until one has worked through the grieving process? People are often aware that the move may reflect an attempt to leave the pain behind.

Only one person in the study was seen at the hospital, and this was at her request. Since this study, and because we offer the facility for people to return and talk to us, many have indeed returned. They are able to discuss the difficulty of walking through the doors into the department again, and returning to the room where their worst fears were confirmed. The opportunity to do this appears to satisfy some need to return to the pain and experience its distress but also to be able to disengage from it.

The respondents were all seen by my colleague Marjorie Ashdown. I had been involved in the immediate care of many of the relatives, and felt that Marjorie would be a more objective listener, and that it would be easier for people to be more openly critical about the experience.

Before she carried out her visit, Marjorie reviewed the nurse's appraisal of the relative's emotional response, and the details of the circumstances of death; these had been elicited by me from nurses within 24 hours of them caring for these relatives. The information obtained at this time included details of who, if anyone, was with the significant relative, and whether they spent time with the deceased. Whether property was taken away immediately, and the total time spent in the department, was also recorded and available to Marjorie.

The average time Marjorie spent listening to each person (or persons) was 3 hours. It is significant that, without exception, everyone said they had never related the whole story before. This became important because the opportunity to review the whole history gave new insights, meaning or understanding of the events, and removed some of the continuing perplexity.

Although the aim of the exercise was to review the events within the hospital, and this was explicitly stated, most people were unable to remain within these parameters. The whole day has major significance, and ends with where and how they slept that night. Consequently, I have since in my bereavement counselling used the question:

'What happened to you on that day?'

Events and interactions both before and after the catastrophe become extremely important.

'I know now, after telling you all this, what I have not done. He never went to work without saying goodbye. It was just another day. I had piles of washing, I remember now. I will hang it out when he has gone to work, I thought.

We valued that time together in a morning. It sounds silly I know. It was really warm and I thought this is stupid, get it out and get it dry. I'm a very practical person, you see.

When I saw his car going out of the gate it annoyed me. He can't even just stop for a moment and say cheerio. I was thinking about him and waiting to say goodbye to him. It never even crossed his mind. Selfish thing, I thought. Typical of men. It sounds stupid now, doesn't it? I have just realized. We never even said goodbye'.

When this lady was called to the hospital, a caring neighbour who accompanied her advised her not to see him when she was told he had died of a heart attack. 'Better remember him as he was,' she said.

She never did get to say goodbye properly. Her review of the whole episode gave her the answer to what was unfinished. She went to the cemetery a week later to do what she now realized she had wanted to do for a long time, to say goodbye. She was also able to express her guilt at feeling annoyed with him as he left her. Once she got this out of the way, she progressed through the other stages of grieving.

Whilst all the issues may not be as clear-cut as that just described, the review of the whole episode deals with the frustration and perplexity surrounding the sequence of events. The impact produces chaos and disorder, and there is a great need to restore order. The review helps to do this.

Several people in our study contacted us again and asked if they could tell it to us all again. Although many of these bereaved people had loving, caring friends and relatives they had not told them the whole story. Listening to the review of events is not only time consuming, it can also be distressing, as can witnessing the grief of the bereaved person. I suspect they were diverted from it, or interrupted, before the story was completed because it was felt to be harmful to them.

In bereavement counselling it may be important that the first session is 2 hours long, to allow a complete review of the day's events. This will often clarify some difficulty, and produce an immediate sense of resolving some issue or changing the focus. It can also highlight any focus of pain. People become fixed on some aspect of the event which appears trivial. This focus grows and becomes an irritation, yet they cannot disengage from it.

Consider the following example: clients are very often angry with themselves for the way some of these peripheral issues take on enormous dimensions.

'When I collected Tom's clothing from the hospital, his jacket was not there. I later found it in the car. Why was he leaving the shop to go to the bank without his jacket on? It was not a very hot day. People must have thought it was odd when they saw him lying there collapsed with no jacket on. He looked smart with it on. If he had been wearing it as usual perhaps he would have been all right. When I picture him lying there without it, it seems all wrong. It is just not him. I just cannot understand why he was without it.'

We eventually progressed to a passer-by having begun cardiac massage and mouth to mouth in an attempt to resuscitate Tom. This led on to the sequence of events culminating in confirmation of his death. This shift of focus was painful and difficult, and led to the widow finally discussing his absence. Her attempts to avoid this had resulted in her preoccupation with some less pertinent aspect. She spent many hours pondering how his death might have been prevented, and somehow the jacket became part of this. She was able, with help, to move on to how life would be for her, without Tom.

The review of the event — a detailed look at the whole day, and how life was prior to and after the death — is time consuming and painful, but may well highlight some difficulty or perplexity previously unresolved. For both client and counsellor confronting the impact of the loss and beginning the process of separation will redefine many issues involved in the process of grieving.

REMEMBERING THE VIGIL

The time of waiting between arrival at the hospital and being given the news of death varies considerably, depending on the cause of death. The difficulties in experiencing extremes of feelings and disordered behaviour, during this period, were described later as torment by people in our study.

If the cause of death is trauma, prolonged measures of intervention in the resuscitation room and then theatre are often undertaken before death occurs. Some patients with serious head injuries may be transferred from another hospital and have a CT scan before theatre. Some time during this evaluation and resuscitation process a patient may die. Patients who arrive in cardiac arrest, having had a heart attack, are often dead on arrival at the hospital, and someone has to make the decision to cease resuscitating them.

Traumatic deaths are likely to be younger people, and our time with the relatives is likely to be longer. The relatives of those who were killed by some outside force, such as a car or a piece of machinery, produce other problems. The deceased is more obviously a victim of someone else. If someone dies of a heart attack and it was felt he brought it on himself because he worked too hard, it is more difficult to blame someone else.

For some relatives, the wait can be up to 2 hours. It may be an hour before they know whether someone is going to live or die, and up to 1 hour in the hospital after they have died. In our study, the longer the experience of not knowing whether the patient would live, the greater the difficulty both at the time and later. The immediate ambivalent feelings were also a difficulty later:

'When waiting to hear if my husband had survived the accident I begged him not to leave me, just to get well. I even threatened him and said don't you dare die now. At the same time I told him I loved him and I could not have found a better husband.

   The awful thing is he did die. I kept going over it all again, pleading with him saying come back, tell me it's all a dream, and then getting angry with him saying he had an absolute nerve to go when we had so much to do. Between this I told him I was sorry I had not told him enough that I loved him. It was so frustrating, going round this thing in this way all the time. You must think I'm mad. I'm not, am I?'

There is obvious difficulty, then, in suddenly experiencing the question of will he live or die, as opposed to the statement 'He is dead.'

'They just said I am sorry he is dead. Just like that. The end. I got up and said, "Well, that's it then. Shall I go home? What do I do now?" There is no way you can argue with the fact that someone is just dead.'

Whilst some people may slip into denial, the clear fact of death leaves no room at the time for negotiating anything else. The statement is final. It is the end.

A sudden death from a heart attack or other medical cause is difficult to come to terms with, but sudden traumatic death is even more so. Obvious ambivalent feelings and disruptive distress and disorder were still apparent at both the 6 month and 10 month period of follow up in our study. This group also described more disruption and difficulties in family relationships. The cot death and the suicide families also identified many issues to explore and clarify, and powerful difficulties in relationships.

People who became very disordered in their behaviour, or displayed marked ambivalence in the immediate time around the death, were showing signs of this later in our study. At the time of the death, it would be useful if we could predict who would later be at risk physically and emotionally. Knowing who would need the most support might prevent long-term damage and breakdown in relationships.

Traumatic, suicide and cot deaths seem to leave people with particularly distressing problems. Most of the people referred to me in my capacity as a bereavement counsellor fit into these groups. Many of the issues arising later reflect difficulties that were apparent in the hospital or at the time of the death, but were not worked with appropriately or easily. Where people in our study had exhibited a clear emotional response in the immediate situation, such as anger or denial, this was still an emotion they were continuing to work with or have difficulty with. It appeared that it was not only the immediately expressed emotional response which was a later issue, but also how it was responded to and worked with.

One lady, seen 6 months after her husband's death on the rugby field at 39 years of age, said:
'First of all can I apologise to you? You must think I was awful. I am not really that sort of person. When I saw him just lying there dead that day, I was so mad. I said, "You bastard, you have left me to bring up three kids alone."

I actually hit him. He had been out enjoying himself and ended up dead. Do you know, I actually hit him on his chest. Tell that nurse I am sorry I embarrassed him. It's funny, because he said, "Don't worry about that. You have every right to be angry, left in the position you are in."

Later, when I felt angry, I did not feel bad about it. As the nurse said, "Who wouldn't with what's happened to you today." '

It was important to this lady that someone in the immediate situation was able to affirm her reaction. Her guilt about her response could have been destructive. Instead, she was able to acknowledge she had needs of her own. This is particularly difficult for women who are told:

'Take care of the kids'
'Be strong for them'
'His mother will need your help and support'

In this case, despite being told all that, she was able to accept her guilt in a useful way and ask for things for herself.

PACTS ABOUT DEATH

Some couples or families will have discussed how they would prefer the partner to respond or cope on the death of one of them and particularly who would 'go first' and what the implications of that might be. This is often discussed at the time of death.

'I should be grateful for her sake that it's her and not me to go now. She always said she wouldn't manage on her own and she wouldn't. For that reason, I should be thankful that this is how it is.'

This person may find it difficult to sustain that thankfulness, and to reconcile it with his grief and despair.

Some of the wishes imposed upon our loved ones regarding death can result in distressing and difficult problems and may damage the remaining partner. If this is raised at the time of death, we may be able to talk about the problem and its potentially damaging aspect.

'He always said I wasn't to grieve for him when he had gone. We had a long and happy life together. We had so much to be thankful for. All sorts of awful things happen to people, they get divorced or have affairs, or end up out of work. Well, nothing like that ever happened to us. He said that whoever went first we were just to think of the good times we had together, and be thankful that nothing terrible ever happened to us. He wouldn't have wanted to see me distressed like this.'

This sort of condition on how to respond to death can be extremely powerful. To have to control one's grief, despair and sense of loss, because of a previously imposed wish, causes many problems. It is obviously done with the best of intentions, as no one would like to visualize their loved ones grieving, and their hope for them would no doubt be that they would recover quickly. We need the process of grief to heal us and allow us to re-emerge from the power of our loss. To ask someone not to grieve is wrong. It is taking away their opportunity to recover.

I find it useful, when spending a longer period with someone at the time of death to ask: 'Did you ever discuss the possibility of this happening?' This gives the opportunity to discuss last wishes and how they are not always useful. Some people will need permission not to adhere to them, and as helpers are sometimes seen as being in authority we may be able to release them from a pact. In working with a long-term difficulty, this issue can often be the key to facilitating the process of grieving.

SUICIDE

For people bereaved by a suicide, 'who was to blame?' either preoccupies them or is carefully avoided. A major assumption is that someone must be to blame. The relatives we saw in our study were extremely anxious about how the material would be used, and whether they were doing the right thing confronting the problem. The issue is either taboo, or one that produces hostility and breakdown in relationships. They often feel it is best avoided, unless blame can be apportioned to their satisfaction.

Evidence collected by Henley (1983) showed that death by suicide results in a bereavement more devastating than any other form of death. In particular, the negative social reactions towards surviving relatives and spouses have serious consequences. Lack of emotional support and practical assistance was a striking factor in Henley's study and she describes a strong avoidance of communication regarding the suicide.

Finding a focus for the fault is not simple, since many factors will have influenced the eventual outcome. Helpers should not collude with the idea of finding the key, the answer to it all. We should be aware that our reaction may be coloured by a particular school of thought. Freud (1917) described the death drive as inherent in all people, in a constant struggle with the will to live. This, he said, accounts for the ambivalence in suicidal

people. Durkheim (1951) considered that suicide is related to the socio-
economic climate.

The cause often occupies and envelops those who have been bereaved
by suicide, and will not go away. It would obviously be a great relief if the
cause could be located and then neatly put away somewhere. Those
bereaved by suicide particularly value the counselling they receive, and
they will need immediate help.

One evening several years ago, a man returned to me very distressed. He
was sent back to the hospital because his family did not know what to do with
him. He was inconsolable.

'This morning, I went round to my brother's house because I had not seen
him for a few days. He lived alone and had bouts of depression. He was a
very private solitary sort of man but he had told me I was his best friend. That
was hard for him to say.

We had a lot in common. We didn't have to say it but we both loved each
other and had an understanding. I had recently gone through a divorce. He
listened, and understood how bad things had been for me. The rest of the
family commented on how we looked after each other. "You are the only one
to get near him," they said.

Over the past week he had been a bit miserable. He sometimes went like
that and sort of hibernated for a week, and I would go round and cheer him up
if I could. I had a key to his house. I was the only one allowed to. He trusted
me.

When I unlocked the door and walked into the hall I thought there was a
funny smell. Then I saw him. It was grotesque, unbelievable, he was hanging
from the banister. He looked horrible. He was clearly dead and I wanted to run
up to him and hold him and shout: No. Why? You'll be all right. Don't, please.
The other part of me made me run, I ran out of the house and fell to the
ground, unable to speak. I thought I was choking.

There were people standing over me looking down, and I thought: In a
minute I will wake up from this horrible nightmare. An ambulance came and
they laid me on a stretcher and carried me into it. It was all real: You are
awake, I told myself, It is all real. I started to shake and then cry, and I could
not stop.

When they took me home from the hospital my parents, brother and sisters
said: "He has taken it very hard." Taken it hard, for God's sake, what do they
expect? They said I should talk to you because I couldn't speak. Well, here I
am talking away without stopping.

It was when they said "He has taken it hard." If I had spoken then they
would not have known what hit them. Yes, I have taken it hard. He said he
loved me and I was his only friend. He knew I had a key and would find him
like that. How can anyone do that to someone?

I hate him. He was a liar to say I was his only friend. You don't do that to friends. I hate the swine and I hope he rots in hell. I will never recover from this, ever. How could you?

Yes, they were right to say I couldn't speak, because if I had they would have heard something they didn't like. How could I do that to my mother. Now I am bad, a wicked person, hating my poor sad brother. What a mess, what an absolute mess.'

He cried for a long time and I held him, and he returned several times to become reconciled to his beloved brother. This reconciliation, even after death, allowed him to begin to live again without him.

As you will appreciate from the above incident, there are many issues to work through, and their avoidance can prevent progress through the grief process. Opportunity must be given to deal with the immense and irrational guilt which is invariably a problem.

The behaviour of the deceased before the suicide has often caused severe relationship difficulties, so life prior to the death has usually been very stressful. This long period of stress, compounded by the suicide, is one of the most traumatic events a person could possibly have to cope with.

Whilst suicide is an intentional act performed by a person to end their own life, there are other types of self-destruction. Other sudden deaths may contain an element of self-destruction, and the bereaved may need further help in confronting this. If self-destruction is apparent at the time of the death, it will be an issue in the later stages of grieving. Overeating, smoking, working too hard, hazardous sports or hobbies or reckless driving may all result in untimely death. Even if you are not working with definite suicide, the contribution of people to their own death could be a counselling point. Relatives left in the immediate throes of the loss may well express anger about this:

'Why did he work so hard? He drove himself to this. The doctor told him to stop smoking but he wouldn't. He has only himself to blame.'

'He knew that racing would kill him one day. He almost expected it. What does that say about him and me?'

The feeling that relatives have in some way been devalued by the deceased, is painful to deal with. In our study, there was evidence that this difficulty was confronted at the time of death, and remained an area to be explored when we saw them later.

Not only is death by suicide untimely, but there are cultural taboos and religious difficulties which can prevent or inhibit expressions of grief. The other ingredients of ambivalence, particularly associated with the pre-death stress, are a mixture of relief and sadness.

Most people bereaved by suicide feel abandoned to sort out this mess, and devalued by the deceased. In my opinion, suicide always needs some counselling support. It would take a very competent, capable individual to handle the psychological difficulties alone.

VIEWING THE BODY

When relatives were seen later in our study they talked of the definite value of contact with the deceased. Viewing the body is especially valued by relatives not present at the point of death. The chance to say 'I am sorry I was not with you,' and to affirm the death, was later described as providing comfort. Also the place where they saw the deceased was commented upon later.

Our study revealed that it is important to see the deceased where they died. This may be a resuscitation room or treatment room. Some saw the body again later, in the chapel next to the hospital mortuary, but said they were most comforted by being able to see them where they had died. This seems to take the bereaved person closer to the event, which they have a strong need to feel part of. There was not one negative response to viewing the body.

When Marjorie Ashdown and I did a phone-in on local radio about sudden death, most of the problems related concerned the absence of a body. One lady rang to say her son was lost overboard at sea 20 years ago, and she still expected him to walk through the door. Wives of pilots missing in the war talked of their difficulty at not having a body to see and confirm death by.

The debate about bringing the bodies of the dead from the Falklands war back to Britain, highlighted this focus on the deceased's body. Raphael (1986) in her experiences with bereavement, and particularly disaster, pointed out that not being able to see the body contributes to later difficulties. Whilst Cathcart (1988) notes that relatives' reluctance to see the body should be respected, she goes on to say they should be encouraged to view and that photographs should be kept.

I am in favour of our current assertive response to viewing the body. The previous response to the question of 'Should I see the body?' was often a passive one: 'You can if you want to' or 'It is your decision'. I have no hesitation now in saying: 'Yes, I think you should.' We can make it a most natural thing to do: 'I am sure you would want to see him, even if it's only to say goodbye.'

Occasionally I hear of someone regretting seeing the deceased, but this is unusual. More regrets and difficulties arise from not seeing the body, and later it is, of course, too late. The risk of regret seems worth taking when a beneficial outcome is likely.

A study by Jones & Buttery (1981) of relatives of sudden death victims who spent time with the body in the Emergency department, also concluded that the viewing process was helpful. Most people stated that the whole episode seemed like a fantasy or a bad dream, and that the viewing made it a reality. Reality, whilst painful, is more manageable than fantasy. Several people in our study who did not see the body had difficulties with fantasies of how it looked. Fantasies can hold you and are less controllable, whilst reality is preferable and frees you from bizarre and distressing images.

People in our study reported that it was helpful, if for example someone was blue-looking after death, to have had this pointed out before they saw the body. In cases of head and facial injuries one might assume it wiser to prevent someone from seeing the body. This is not so, as long as people are told before going in to view. If necessary the injuries can be covered, and it need not prevent them holding the deceased's hand.

Viewing the body was certainly a major issue in our feedback from relatives. It affirmed for me that the time and effort spent with relatives and the deceased are tremendously valuable. There seems little doubt that it helps to begin the process of grief, and it was important to us as a team, in the Accident & Emergency Department, to have this sort of positive feedback.

THE CONCLUDING TRANSACTION

Relatives also described in our study how they felt, after news of the death was given and they had viewed the body, about having to leave and go home. We have noticed that there is, understandably, a reluctance to leave. How can you leave the person behind? People may need help to leave, and yet should not feel they are being rushed out. One of the anxieties about offering people the opportunity to sit with the body can be that they would not want to leave. This rarely happens, but if it does it should be openly discussed.

Part of the concluding process may be to sign for and take away valuables such as rings or a watch, or signing for and receiving clothing. Information on how to contact the coroner, or obtain a death certificate bring the transaction on to a more practical level. People realize they have to go home and, on a practical level, make arrangements for a funeral or to take up life without the deceased.

People appear to need a clear indication that they can leave. After being asked if there are any questions left unanswered they actually do need permission to leave. No dissatisfaction was expressed about this at follow up in our study.

As a result of our study, we now offer people the facility of returning, either soon or in the longer term, to discuss any outstanding issues. This offer is often accepted. The card given to them with the telephone number of the hospital and the coroner also states the name of the nurse who looked after them so that they can contact this key individual. Careful records need to be kept, as some people may not contact the hospital until a year later. The nurse involved is likely to have retained a great deal of information, but if he or she has left good records are essential.

The relatives' evaluation of how we viewed their emotional response to the loss in our study is explored in more detail in the next chapter. Some of the insights into these responses, gained on retrospective evaluation, help us to feel more comfortable about them. The next chapter identifies the responses that proved most difficult and describes how relatives later felt about their responses. How they viewed our difficulty with them is also important.

Our contact with relatives who agreed to share their experiences of this painful and difficult time has been a great help for evaluating how we can care more effectively for people. For those of us who work with the pain and distress of sudden death, it has validated our efforts and commitment. We have also been reminded that there is much to learn about the process and immediate care, if we choose to listen.

I am often asked if this work is depressing. Hearing of some of the terrible and overwhelming difficulties of people, and how they overcome them, is far from depressing. It highlights the resourcefulness and courage of the bereaved, and the care and support that is available from family and friends, or from professionals.

Activity 3C

Write notes on the most favourable conditions for allowing someone to tell their story.

REFERENCES

Bayliss M 1994 My long road to Japan. Unpublished story
Cathcart F 1988 Seeing the body after death. British Medical Journal 297:997–998
Durkheim E 1951 Suicide. The Free Press, New York
Freud S 1917 Mourning and melancholia, standard edn, vol. XIV. Hogarth, London
Henley S 1983 Bereavement by suicide. Bereavement Care, vol. 2, Cruse, London
Huelskoetter M M W, Murray R B 1991 Psychiatric/mental health nursing. Appleton & Lange, Connecticut
Jones W H, Buttery M 1981 Sudden death — survivors' perceptions of their emergency department experience. Journal of Emergency Nursing 7:1
Jung K 1961 Memories, dreams and reflections. Vintage, New York
McKechnie R 1993 Earwitness to disaster. Journal of Accident & Emergency Nursing 1(3):149–153
Picard C 1990 Caring and the story. In: D Gaunt (ed.) Caring—the compassionate healer. NLN, New York
Raphael B 1986 When disaster strikes. Hutchinson, London

The death of a child

A child is many things: a part of self and of the loved partner; a representation of the generations past; the genes of the forebears; the hope of the future; a source of love, pleasure, even narcissistic delight; a tie or a burden; and sometimes a symbol of the worst part of the self and others.

Beverley Raphael 1984

The death of a child will be a complex and painful life event. The death does not fit into the natural order of things. Rando (1985) writes that parents feel it is unnatural that the child predeceases them. The role of providing for, guiding and doing things for the child is central to a parent's identity.

A bereaved parent has feelings of helplessness, failure and guilt, and the death of a child will have major consequences for the health and well-being of the bereaved. Parkes (1975) identifies the determinants of an unfavourable outcome and how deaths preceded by little warning have serious implications for the recovery process.

Parental distress is increased by separation from the child (Renner 1991). The sudden nature of the death may mean one or both parents were not present at the time of the death. Regrets about this continually overwhelm the bereaved in the grieving process. Even when many other issues have been dealt with in counselling, this one will not go away. The parents feel they have failed the child by not being present. Measures can sometimes be taken to prevent this happening, for example by making the child more accessible during resuscitation and at the time of and after death.

Another cause for regret may be that parents did not see the child's body. This can also have a strong influence on the grieving process.

Intervention by Accident & Emergency department staff will have a significant impact on the parents' grief response (Parrish et al 1987). Most parents who viewed their dead child's body in our study agreed that, though painful, viewing did create a strong sense of the reality of the death. The decision to view did not appear to have any relation to cause of death (medical or traumatic). It is likely that reducing the number of people with regrets would have a positive influence on perceived care.

Staff should deal proactively with the question of whether children present should view the dead child's body. If asked by the family whether a child should do so, a neutral position should be taken, and a discussion on the merits of doing so can take place. It is an area where the family could be in conflict, often holding opposite views.

The family will value the help of an objective outsider (staff) in helping them arrive at a decision about viewing. Staff should be sensitive to people's feelings, however, and especially avoid referring to the deceased in terms of 'the body' or 'it', because this is very upsetting (Dubin & Sarnoff 1986).

If the child's body is damaged the bereaved should be informed, but should not be prevented from spending time with the deceased (Cassem 1978). Staff should clean and make the child's body as presentable as possible.

A study of 81 parents whose child had died suddenly reported that nearly all of them wished to spend time with the dead child, even when the body was mutilated (Finlay & Dallimore 1991). Of the 81, 49 felt they had not been given enough time with the child, particularly when the death had been caused by a road traffic accident, and 2 of the parents in this study remained angry that they had been actively dissuaded from seeing their child's body. Several expressed regret that they were not allowed to hold, wash or touch the child after death.

This study also indicated that 68% of these parents had not been approached about organ donation. Of this group, 59% wished they had been approached, which suggests that the option of organ donation may help rather than hinder the parents' grief process.

Many studies stress the importance of the parents knowing they can return and spend time with the dead child. Parents often have other family members with whom they wish to return to the child.

Written details given on leaving about whom to contact for further information, ongoing help and support is valued. Lack of more formal support from community services has been criticized (Rostron 1981). Lundin (1984) reported an increased psychiatric morbidity in a sample of relatives after sudden unexpected deaths. All the indications are that most parents will benefit from some ongoing counselling, and from access to the health care staff involved at the time of their child's death. The immediate care will have a profound influence on the whole process of grief when a child has died.

Activity 4A

Make a list of community resources available for bereaved parents.

Jane was sitting alone in the relatives' room when I walked in. It would be better to describe her as crouching with her arms wrapped round herself. She rubbed and squeezed her arms and body, and the anguish was apparent on her face.

'He is dead, isn't he?'

Just 15 minutes before, her only baby son had arrived in an ambulance, lifeless. The resuscitation measures had just been abandoned. There was clearly no hope on arrival, and he appeared to have been dead for some time. After this was established, and as we were discussing the baby as being a victim of 'cot death', I was interrupted. 'His mother has arrived,' were the words that quickly shifted our thoughts to the distress of the child's mother.

John, her husband, was driving down separately, and Jane had sat in the front of the ambulance as it sped through the streets, siren wailing and blue light flashing. Jane's whole posture and overwhelming sadness were visibly apparent. There was no hope, no request for him to be spared, no denial of the awful reality. She knew. My nod of the head and hoarse 'Yes' confirmed what she least wanted to know. She cried and held my hand, and inattentively stroked my arm, her thoughts elsewhere.

'You won't leave me, will you? Where is John?'

She quickly filled me in on Adam's short life, assuring me he was loved and wanted, and how in the 12 weeks he was alive he had begun to thrive and have a personality of his own. One idea had been that he might be a musician. What a great gift, she said, to make people happy with music.

'I must have done something really wicked to deserve this. How stupid not to notice he might be ill or sickening for something.'

The reassurances that this happens without warning or symptoms, and how we believed he was the victim of sudden infant death syndrome afforded little apparent consolation.

The paediatrician arrived, and told Jane how our immediate efforts to find signs of life had produced nothing, confirming that when Jane found Adam at home he had been dead. He went on to tell her what we knew about sudden infant death syndrome, and told her he would send for both Jane and her husband in 5 weeks' time to discuss it again.

When the doctor left we realized that John had not arrived, and soon afterwards a phone call from a neighbouring hospital informed us that he had arrived there; in his turmoil, Jane's big, strong man had rushed to the wrong place.

'That's not like him,' Jane said. 'Quiet, strong and well organized. Poor John, he didn't know what to do with me or himself.'

John's guilt at getting to the wrong hospital and not being present to comfort Jane was soon verbalized on his arrival. He held her whilst she cried loudly and painfully. (Such a cry that once you have heard it you know what it means.) I explained to them that I would arrange for them to see Adam, and how they would both have much to say and reflect upon together with him. Jane said at once:

'Yes, take me to him now.'

I left them together, explaining I would need to check that everything was ready for them to see Adam. As I was leaving the room, John turned to a very fragile looking Jane, sat her on his knee and held her to him.

Adam was, by now, in a clean baby gown and wrapped in a blanket. The staff had taken a great deal of pride in seeing that he looked just right for his parents and someone had put a single flower in his hand. Jane, well supported by John, entered the room and immediately both of them began to cry loudly. Jane lifted Adam up and cradled him in her arms and her anger and distress were painful:

'Why have you left me and hurt me in this way?' she asked
'Please come back, come back'
'Wake him up, please,' she begged me.

'I wish I could,' were all the words I could muster, and John looked at me pleadingly:

'Please help her, please.'

He looked around helplessly, and this strong grown man began to shake and thump the palm of his hand in his frustration and helplessness. He was so used to putting things right for his wife. Jane was by now walking up and down, holding Adam tightly to her.

'Can we take him home, John, and just bury him in the garden?'
'No, Jane you can not,' John replied. 'Tell her not to say that.'

Her thoughts were elsewhere and John began to shake and cry. Jane was now sitting, holding her baby.

'I am sorry,' John said, 'please let me go outside, I need some air.'

I left the room with him. He stood shaking and looked ready to explode with the grief. 'You want to be strong for Jane', I said. 'But who would be a Dad at times like this. Dads feel pain, feel grief and feel helpless. Who looks after you?' He held on to me and wept bitterly, and I held him. Nothing was said for at least 5 minutes and then he put into words exactly what was happening.

'I need so much to hold on to you and for you to hold on to me.'

This was the acknowledgement that he had both these needs and he was giving himself permission to have them.

We returned to the room and Jane was sitting quietly, rocking to and fro more peacefully. I explained that Adam was in a hospital nightdress and that they might feel better if he was wearing his 'best' clothes or something of his own. He may have a favourite toy that they would like him to have close to him.

We began to talk of grandparents, aunts and uncles, close friends, and the need to inform them. Jane and John were both assured that all were free to come and see Adam in the Chapel of Rest if they wished. Jane particularly was advised that she and John were free to return day and night within the first few days, and was warned gently that she might wake in the night and wonder where he was. It was important that at times like these she should know where she could come and see him.

Whilst the last thing in the world she wanted was confirmation of where he was, this is, in my experience, preferable to not being able to see him. The hours of the night are long and lonely, and using this period to hold the baby and reflect can offer some comfort. Jane said she knew she would have to take me up on the offer.

After I had spent some time explaining the involvement of the coroner and the need for a postmortem, they prepared to leave. Literature from the Foundation for the Study of Infant Deaths was handed to them, with written details of my name and telephone number. As they left, both said they might possibly need to return and talk, and John said, half smiling:

'I may need you to cry with again.'

Both did return, on several occasions. Over the next 2 or 3 days, they called and sat and held Adam in the hospital chapel. His favourite toy elephant was brought, his bright red suit and his only lace-up shoes, that Jane felt so good about putting on his feet.

His grandparents, aunts and uncles came, some together, some alone. In Jane's periods alone with Adam, she was sometimes angry and remonstrated with him for leaving her, and then was angry with herself for loving him too much. One morning, when John said he knew how she felt, she protested loudly that he had never been Adam's mother.

Both decided on the fourth day that they would not visit after the postmortem. They sat alone with Adam and said final goodbyes. As Jane handed him back to me that night she said:

'I know this is it now. He cannot be with me any longer.'

They quickly said goodbye and left. As they walked out, I thought of all we had achieved together, and yet knew this was only the beginning.

Jane and John did not respond to our request to take part in the study. The feedback I received was over a year later, when Jane asked to see me. She described much love and support from John and their family and friends, and her involvement in a group for 'cot-death mothers'. She valued the sharing of experiences and the support this group gave her.

She had returned to give me two messages. One was to say they were slowly emerging from this 'and from time to time you must have a need to know this.' How right she was! Secondly she wanted to say how much she had valued that immediate care, and that she now realized how much work she had done at the time. The word 'work' was hers. She described her confrontation with death, with its awful reality. She then recalled her unhurried opportunity to reflect on Adam's short life in the presence of his death. This confrontation with death's reality, and her realistic perception of the event, clearly ties in with one of the three components of crisis intervention that we have to work with.

The moment Jane found most significant was, in many respects, the most painful. She recalled how she handed the baby back to me, having arrived at the decision not to see his body again. She told me how important it was to finally feel able to do that:

'I did so much work in those 3 days to be able to arrive at that moment.'

She described how she had come to realize this from her encounters with other mothers who had experienced cot deaths. Some had not been given the opportunity to work in this way in the immediate situation, or were prevented from doing so by themselves or other well-meaning people. She described herself and the others who had responded and worked in the immediate situation as being months and maybe years ahead in the process of grieving.

It was clear to Jane that the immediate input in the hospital had begun that process we call grief, and had allowed her to re-emerge from the distress it caused. She had done this sooner than the others who were not given the same opportunities or freedom to encounter death; their ambivalent feelings and distress, although painful, were then encountered again and again, and the difficulties of denial were less apparent.

Jane confirmed for me what many other parents of 'cot death' babies have said. At the immediate time of the loss, and on subsequent days, the bereaved parents must be given one or more key workers and several hours to talk through the loss and to encounter the dead baby as frequently as they wish.

The opportunity to deal with the feelings of anger as well as grief, and talk through all the details of the death, is tremendously important. Time to reflect on the life of the baby, and on the nature of the relationship with parents and others, is the beginning of a recurrent need to review the details of the death.

SUDDEN INFANT DEATH SYNDROME

Where there has been a 'cot death', the bereaved parents have some obvious and apparent needs. Difficulty with the reality of the death, and confronting the death, will be a problem for both the parents and the care workers. Ambivalence about what to do will compound this difficulty.

An apparently healthy baby is put to sleep in a cot or pram. Occasionally the baby has some minor symptoms. These may be a snuffly nose, or perhaps he did not take as much feed as he normally would. When next looked at, the baby is dead. This is slightly more common in boys than in girls, and more frequent in winter months. In the UK about one baby in every 500 live births dies suddenly and unexpectedly. In many parts of the world it is the most common cause of death in the age group of 1 month to 1 year.

When later examined by a pathologist, a small number of these babies revealed a previously unsuspected abnormality or an overwhelming infection. In the majority of cases, however, death is difficult or impossible to explain. In the absence of any known cause these deaths will be registered as sudden infant death syndrome. With present knowledge the death cannot be foreseen by parents or doctors. Most of the babies will die silently in their sleep or if not asleep rapidly become unconscious and die. There is no indication they suffer distress or pain. Those found face down or covered with a blanket may cause parents to think they suffocated and that they are to blame. External suffocation, however, is not the cause of sudden infant death syndrome.

Sometimes vomit is found around the mouth or on the bedclothes. This will lead to the conclusion that the baby choked on his vomit or his last feed. Many parents bemoan the fact that they did not spend enough time with the baby or 'getting his wind up' after a feed. The presence of vomit occurs during or after a death and is not in itself a cause of death in these babies.

When a normal baby dies there just has to be an answer, it must be explained. In the immediate situation questions about the cause may be repeated time and time again. The search for an answer inevitably leads parents to ask who is to blame. Parents can blame themselves, the doctor, the health visitor, the baby sitter, and frequently God.

Over half of sudden infant death syndrome babies arrive in Emergency departments. The apparently overwhelming grief and distress may cause the ambulance personnel to bring the baby to hospital alone. They have a need to remove the pain (the dead baby) from the parents, or they may not have had time to wait for the parents in their urgency to resuscitate the baby. Parents may not have been able to leave other children who are at home. When they ring the hospital later, both parents should be invited to come to the hospital as soon as possible. This may be resisted if someone knows the baby is dead. A typical response may be:

'Is there any point in bringing the mother?'
'Can you just confirm the baby is dead?'

Many times both parents will arrive and, when death has been confirmed, will want to see and hold the baby. The role of the coroner's officer (policeman, applies to England and Wales only) will need to be explained. It is important that as much information as possible is imparted, to deal with their helplessness and perplexity.

Care workers will need to explain that other relatives, such as grand-parents, may want to see the baby and they must feel free to bring them along. The offer of open access to the dead baby prior to postmortem is important. It is important that the parents are not left alone unless they request it, and that they have the opportunity to review the whole of the event prior to departure. The arrival of the other significant people in their lives will allow them to re-live the events. This process, often called the 'obsessional review' will be a major part of the ongoing grieving process.

If the mother is breast-feeding, she will need immediate practical advice on the suppression of lactation. Written information to take away with them, on what we know about SIDS and on obtaining further help, is available from the Foundation for the Study of Infant Deaths (the address appears in the appendix).

All clothing removed from the baby should be placed in separate bags for collection by the coroner's officer. This includes soiled clothing and nappies. Nothing should be discarded or destroyed. Although the baby may have been placed in a clean gown, the parents can be offered the opportunity of returning with the child's own clothes and maybe a favourite toy.

The absence of a definite cause of death gives rise to guilt and to blame. Other people's response will compound this; they too will be perplexed, questioning and puzzled. In the absence of a reasonable explanation people may resort to fantasy: 'Somebody did something wrong'. Every little detail will be examined and some inconsequential aspect is often seized upon. The search for answers is relentless, and drains parents of all resources.

Another difficulty is that for legal reasons the sudden death will be carefully investigated. The questioning of all involved, from emergency services, hospital staff and the coroner's officer is often interpreted as an accusation of neglect.

Tensions between couples are often apparent at the time of the death. Consequent ambivalence and lack of sexual intimacy for fear of further pregnancy and loss can put the relationship at risk.

The postmortem may be perceived as a further violation of this innocent child. Having failed to prevent the death, the parents will then be angry about failing to prevent this. It all compounds their helplessness and the loss of their parental role. When the postmortem result is available the parents should be given every opportunity to discuss its contents.

Siblings of the dead child should not be overlooked. Grief-stricken parents may not be able to deal with difficult questions from other children. Siblings' previous ambivalence about this baby can result in feelings of guilt and responsibility for the death. Problems at school and with sleeping are common in these children.

MISCARRIAGE

A miscarriage is also a death of a child, though this is often overlooked. Because we are concerned for the mother's health, the loss or grief might be missed. Focusing on future pregnancies may be a way of dealing with the present loss.

The woman who has experienced a miscarriage will have the added anxiety of whether future pregnancies are possible at all. Some causes will have a clear medical explanation, others will not. Again, there is a relentless search for explanation. In the absence of a satisfactory explanation the woman often blames herself, sometimes focusing on too much strenuous activity or work. Her partner's need or her need for continuing sexual activity can make him a target for the blame.

There is a need to grieve the loss of this little person. As others outside the immediate circle of family are often unaware of the loss there may be less opportunity to talk about it.

Rituals (funerals) can be arranged for fetuses of all ages, and parents need to be offered the opportunity for this. Many women I have counselled after a sudden death have the added problem of a previous loss re-emerging and compounding the present one. This previous loss is often a miscarriage with no opportunity to mourn for the baby.

Of course the loss is not only the mother's, it also affects the father, other siblings, family and friends. Despite remarks being made to the contrary, many mums say of this tiny baby 'I was beginning to get to know him.'

STILL BIRTHS

The response of a mother and father at this crisis is similar to other child deaths: anger, loss, guilt and questioning. 'What have I done wrong? Why me?' The important role of the staff at the start of this grief work remains the same. The parents are also aware of disappointing many others who are waiting for this baby: parents, siblings, other children within the family. Not only have parents not received what they wanted, but they also failed to provide this baby for others.

Any ambivalence previously experienced about the pregnancy will carry guilt into the grieving process, and affect self-esteem. Thoughts will dwell on the idea that for some reason they deserved this.

Some deaths at birth will be known about before the event. It is particularly distressing to have to wait for the onset of labour to produce a dead baby. Although you would expect some anticipatory grieving the awful reality has still to be confronted. Most mothers are anxious to see, touch and hold the baby, whilst some fathers may want to prevent this.

Some people will want photographs of the dead baby to confirm evidence of the pregnancy and that it produced a baby. There is a danger that the parents will feel the whole experience was unreal. Raphael (1984) highlights how many women are heavily sedated through the still birth experience and afterwards. This may prevent them from seeing the baby and also suppress the grieving response.

It is essential to care for both parents, involving them in the rituals and actualizing the loss (Wordon 1991). Couples are not only grieving for what they have lost but also for what they might have had.

ABORTION

When counselling someone in grief over the death of a child or fetus, I am no longer surprised if a previous abortion compounds their current difficulty. At this stage it is often clear to the sufferer that they failed to mourn the previous loss. There will be many reasons for this. It is the unspeakable loss. It is difficult to grieve for the child when you made the decision to terminate the pregnancy.

One immediate response to the termination could be relief, and this is difficult to integrate with loss and grief. To focus on 'the child' is painful; it makes him or her 'real', with an identity. It is easier to depersonalize the child, in order to dilute or displace the pain.

The later grief I have shared with parents who have experienced thera-peutic abortion has emphasized their need to grieve and the impossibility of doing so. Some people perceive further deaths or losses as a punish-ment. It is therefore important to work with the impact. This remains a very difficult task.

SOME FINAL REMARKS

Not all children are babies or young adults. A 'child' may have been an autonomous adult, leading a life independent of parents for many years. If this child dies it is still the 'wrong order of things'. An often-heard remark from an elderly parent focuses on this: 'It should have been me. It is my turn.' This can lead to bargaining and heavenward glances: 'Take me instead of him' or 'I wish there was some way you could swap us around.' Often there are discussions on the nature of relationships:

'He was my first'
'We had this special affinity'
'She was always close to me'

This most traumatic experience of child death produces feelings of isolation in parents. Many tell me they feel no one could get near or understand the depth of their distress. Often they are angry that this is even suggested to them. They experience feelings of self-blame and often a need for revenge (Weinberg 1994). The preliminary findings in Weinberg's study have implications for bereavement work and emphasize the difficulty of working through these feelings. The death of a child is a powerful confrontation with the fact that we are not in control of children's lives.

Activity 4B

Discuss or write what you think will be the differences in response to the death of a child:
1. in a road traffic accident
2. because of a therapeutic abortion.

REFERENCES

Cassem N H 1978 Treating the person confronting death. In: Nicholi A M (ed) The Harvard guide to modern psychiatry. Belknap Press of Harvard University Press, Massachusetts
Dubin W R, Sarnoff J R 1986 Sudden and unexpected death — interventions with the survivors. Annals of Emergency Medicine 15(1):54–57
Finlay I, Dallimore D 1991 Your child is dead. British Medical Journal 302:1524–1525
Lundin T 1984 Morbidity following sudden and unexpected bereavement. British Journal of Psychiatry 144:84–88
Parkes C M 1975 Determinants of outcome following bereavement. Omega (Journal of Death & Dying) 6(4):303–323
Parrish G A, Holden K S, Skiendzielewski J J 1987 Emergency department experience with sudden death: a survey of survivors. Annals of Emergency Medicine 16:792–796
Rando T A 1985 Bereaved parents: particular difficulties, unique factors and treatment issues. Social Work 30(1):19–23
Raphael B 1984 The anatomy of bereavement. Hutchinson, London
Renner S 1991 I desperately needed to see my son. British Medical Journal 302:356
Rostron J 1981 The needs of the family following a fatal road traffic accident. Public Health 95:353–355
Weinberg N 1994 Self blame, other blame and desire for revenge: factors in recovery from bereavement. Death Studies 18:583–593
Wordon W 1991 Grief counselling and grief therapy. Routledge, London

5

The suddenly bereaved child

My eyes searched my mum's face. It couldn't be true. I didn't want it to be true but my mum's pale face told me it was true. I cried. It broke my heart. I had lost my brother. I had just lost my faith in the world. How could it be so cruel to a happy 10 year old girl who had never done anything wrong? This was the summer the world betrayed me.

Madeleine Rigby, 1994

Since writing the first edition of this book I have been part of an almost weekly clinic for bereaved children. The families of the children, and occasionally the children themselves, have sought help with a sudden death.

I have sometimes met the children previously, at the time of the sudden death, often when I and a member of their family or a close friend have told them about the death of a loved one. Children are great and profound teachers and over the years they have taught me much about childhood loss. Their openness and honesty is wonderful, and a great problem to adults.

Childhood is often romanticized by adults. They think of children as being part of a protected world where their needs are met and where they are safe and untainted. Yet even in the best of worlds a child lives with inner uncertainty and fear.

Adults will talk of the time this innocent world is shattered by introducing issues about sex and, that other dreaded event, death.

'They are too young'
'They do not need to know about that, not yet'
'They will not understand'
'It is too much to contemplate'.

It hurts us to see the dream shattered, the story spoiled. Children seem too young to be contaminated by death; they will learn about it soon enough.

If the death is expected, parents and families will hopefully prepare children for the inevitable. With sudden death the possible responses of a child to the news include:

- shock and disbelief
- dismay and protest
- apathetic, stunned, withdrawn
- continues with usual activities.

Shock and disbelief. Children will often say 'It can't be true' or 'I don't believe you', and for a while they will maintain this:

'Tell me this is a dream'
'Say he will come back'
'It is a mistake. Tell me you are wrong'.

Dismay and protest. 'Don't say that', 'Be quiet', 'It's not fair', 'I want him back' are common responses. At the same time the child may lash out in anger at the bearer of the message: 'I hate you', 'Go away'.

Apathetic, stunned withdrawn. There is little or no response here but the child is clearly hurt. They look uncomprehending and perplexed. They may look around puzzled, and suggest by their expression that it all seems unreal. The bearer of the news may wonder whether they should repeat it, or check that it has been understood.

Continues with usual activities. 'Can I go home now?', 'When can I go out and play?', 'I want everyone to stop crying and be happy again', are responses that suggest flight or denial and a need to return to normal.

BREAKING THE NEWS

Ideally the news of the death should be given by a parent or close family member. However, these people also are bereaved, rendered helpless, incapacitated by the whole event. They will feel they have little or no resources for themselves, and the task may overwhelm them. I feel we should offer to help them break the bad news. The worker who is adamant that only family should do this may be saying this because the thought of it overwhelms them emotionally. It can be an attempt at avoidance. I have worked with many families who have been helped to break the bad news to children, and they are clear about how much they valued this support and help.

How should we say it; where to begin; what words should we use; how will we deal with it? These are all questions that highlight the over-whelming nature of the task of breaking bad news.

Children should not be kept waiting for long or be told to occupy themselves for a while. They are very perceptive; they know something terrible has occurred and will be frightened by lack of information. The presence of many people in the room will overwhelm children and produce a multifaceted response when they are given the news. It is better to have one or two people, depending on the number of children, and a quiet, private place.

Initially, the information should be short, clear and unambiguous (Grollmann 1992): 'I have some bad news for you. Your mummy has died.' After the initial response has been dealt with, more information can be given if the request for further information is not part of the response: 'She was driving to work today, was in an accident and died from the injuries (or damage to her).'

After the initial outpouring of feelings, more information is usually demanded. I have found that too much information is not easily processed. Children's own questions, either initially or over the next few days, will indicate the pace and their ability to gain a greater understanding of the event.

The words 'died' and 'dead' are clear and usually understood. 'Lost' or 'in a long sleep' confuse and produce fears. The child must be kept near to any surviving parent or close relative throughout the waiting period. Sudden offers of help from others, to take the child away to their own house, should be avoided, especially if some distance is involved. Helping children in familiar surroundings provokes less anxiety.

There is a tendency in surviving adults to rescue children from witnessing grief. This isolation from the grief, and keeping them in ignorance of it in order to protect them, causes more problems than it prevents. Children must be allowed to cry (not told to be brave), to scream, be silent or express anger.

It is also important not to quickly dismiss children's expressions of responsibility. Allow this to be verbalized, tell them you understand how they think that, and then explain how the incident occurred. Rapid, bland, dismissive responses do not work.

Many children are unable to sit down when discussing these issues. Some walk around, play with a toy or other object. It is not inappropriate or selfish to have a need of some object or food or drink. These are often a comfort.

VIEWING THE BODY

Children must be allowed to see and, if they wish, to touch the person who has died. They should never be hurried or forced to do so nor made to feel guilty if they do not wish to. What they will see, and what it means, must be explained to them. They must always be accompanied and supported by Accident & Emergency staff, with members of the family if necessary. Above all, they should not be pressurized or rushed but allowed to delay or repeat this final 'saying goodbye'.

When the dead person is disfigured or mutilated the child's wishes about seeing the body are still paramount. Gentle, honest explanations beforehand are crucial. Commensurate with the child's understanding they can inform, but except in extreme circumstances must not influence the child's decision to see the dead person.

Advice to the surviving close adult, about the child's immediate and future needs and possible reactions, is needed. Simple advice notes to take away and share with other adults are more valuable than lengthy immediate verbal advice which will often not be understood or remembered.

INFORMATION FOR OTHERS WHO ARE SIGNIFICANT IN THE CHILD'S LIFE

The GP, school nurse and health visitor, and (if involved) the social worker, will need to know about the bereaved child. It is also important that they know what the child has been told. Inconsistencies in information will add further to the confusion experienced by the child. Try to obtain the parent's consent to talk to the head of the child's school. The school can offer support to the child and the head may decide to disclose some basic details to other children in the class. School staff often regret they were not involved in this way, since their involvement can make a difference to the ensuing distress suffered by the child. Families will need to know where further support would be available for children if this were felt necessary. Whatever sources of help are identified, the vital role of the school should not be underestimated (Capewell 1994).

ASSESSING THE DIFFICULTY FOR EACH CHILD

Childhood bereavement is affected by:

- nature and circumstances of death
- age of child
- gender
- family rules about expression of feeling
- adults' ability to cope
- past experience of loss.

These are outlined in more detail next.

The nature of the death and its circumstances. Here we begin with a difficulty because the death was sudden and the child has had no opportunity to anticipate it. The child will ponder in detail how the person died, whether there was any damage to the person, and whether they suffered and were frightened. These are the very aspects that cause adults great pain, the aspects they do not wish to discuss with the child.

Some adults will simply say that the child must not know, that it would be too difficult to contemplate. Many of the children I have seen have had part of the information already, from listening in to adult conversations. We must consider what words we use and how we will discuss the circumstances with the child.

If there is an inquest and it is reported in the media, school friends may well overhear and then repeat adult conversations about it. If the bereaved child hears the details later, in the school playground, the distress will be far greater.

Age of the child. This will affect the child's perception of the event as follows:

- Below 5 years
  - lack of understanding about the finality of death
  - an inability to run through the events and arrive at a logical conclusion, 'Going round in circles'
  - a belief that they can cause what happens to them and around them — egocentricity.
- 5–10 years
  - concrete thinking, literal understanding
  - understanding the physical causes of death, both internal and external
  - concern with other people's feelings — empathy
  - an interest in the more tangible expressions of grief: rituals, pictures, gravestones.
- 10 years and older
  - a more abstract understanding
  - a great sense of justice/injustice, fate
  - reflection of belief systems
  - strong emotional reaction.

Gender. Boys may be given messages about being strong and in control: 'You are the man of the house now'. From an early age they may have been told about the value of being strong and in control. The girls may be perceived as the ones to overtly express the grief, and as the vehicle to express the whole family's grief. Some girls will be considered as being fragile and may have to cope with limitation of information.

Family rules about expressing feelings. This applies not only to gender but also to the whole family system of expressing emotion. It can be detected at the time of impact, and from the way they respond to each other.

Adults' ability to cope. If the closest adults are having trouble coping, they will have few or no resources for the children.

Past experiences of loss. How previous losses were dealt with (or not dealt with), will influence the child's ability to manage the present crisis. Previous losses may have made the child less or more resourceful.

The above considerations will help us to decide how to offer further help proactively, and will give some insight into the long-term risk to the bereaved child. One longer-term option is to offer the opportunity for children to explore their grief in groups (Davidson–Neilson & Leick 1993, Fell 1994).

Caring for grief-stricken children can be very distressing for adults. The work makes us vulnerable and people working in the field stress the importance of recognizing this (Dyregrov 1990). Debriefing after the immediate care may be needed and ongoing care often requires supervision for the care workers. Counselling for parents or the family involved may be needed in the long term.

Activity 5A

Describe the feelings you may have when confronted with breaking the news of a death to a child. How could these feelings adversely affect the child?

REFERENCES

Capewell E 1994 Responding to children in trauma. Bereavement Care 13(1):2–7
Davidson–Neilson M, Leick N 1993 Directive grief treatment in a group setting. Bereavement Care 12(3):29–32
Dyregrov A 1990 Grief in children. Jessica Kingsley, London
Fell M 1994 Helping older children grieve: a group therapy approach. Health Visitor 67(3):92–94
Grollman E A 1992 Talking about death. Beacon, Boston
Rigby M 1994 The summer the world betrayed me. Bereavement Care 13(3):30–32

The problems of the care worker

Health professionals avidly seek culture through the arts. We welcome the suffering experience expressed in music, the arts, Greek drama and the world's literature. Yet when the suffering patient wishes to express the experience he or she is having, the shared observations are like a foreign language in the health care milieu. And when the patient begins to ask aloud the centuries-old questions — Why me? Why now? Why? — that each of us will ultimately ask, the audience dwindles and slips away. Just as isolation techniques are used to protect the staff from communicable diseases, we protect ourselves by a form of shunning of the patient who attempts to grope verbally for meaning to attach to his or her pain and suffering. What we fear is not a microorganism but rather the confronting of our own mortality or, even worse than death, our own suffering experience.

Laurel Archer Copp 1993

This chapter highlights how easy it is for the worker to become disempowered. Whatever your profession, when caring for the suddenly bereaved you can quickly feel you are not in control. In the interpersonal dynamics of caring this should be a daily consideration. Issues such as domination, control, facilitation, empowerment, helping, enabling, exercise of authority, compliance/submission are all relevant to the ethics of the caring relationship.

In the interaction of breaking bad news and caring for the suddenly bereaved, the pendulum often seems to have swung too far against the worker. In my workshops, the helplessness of the worker is often revealed as painfully overwhelming:

'I felt useless'
'There was nothing I could do'
'There was no way I could put it right.'

In the face of the stark reality of the pain expressed, many workers know they have no alternative but to stay with it. There is no easy answer, no obvious solution, no way of taking control and making it better.

We need to know that our immediate care, and its quality, can have long-term implications in the recovery of individuals. A greater understanding of the emotional responses of those involved in a sudden death can make it all more manageable. For example, certain emotional responses from relatives of sudden death victims are more likely than others to leave the carer distressed or feeling ineffective. From our study we were able to identify what these responses to immediate news of a sudden death were, so that they could be looked at more closely.

Despite our knowledge of these responses and insight into the process of grieving, we nevertheless have to make contact with the raw feelings, and this will be painful. That hurt, that encounter with grief on its impact, is very distressing and disruptive, and we have to cope with the disorder that results. Some insights into what can leave us feeling ineffective, or into what lies behind this response in the relative, can help the carer. It somehow lessens feelings of chaos and disorder if we can identify the response either at the start of or during the process of grieving.

The primary focus of this chapter is what incapacitates the carer, but how the clients felt about their immediate response at a later date will also be considered. The emotional stance a client takes on impact, the particular response that emerges, or how he defends himself at this time, can give some insight into the person and his struggles with the grief. Whilst responses are not to be judged right or wrong, some need more working with immediately and are less well dealt with by the person from whom they emerge. A response that makes a carer uncomfortable may be beneficial to the client, whilst responses that carers find acceptable or easier to manage could create difficulty for the client; crying is the only response that both client and carer tend to feel comfortable with.

Another result that emerged from our study was that the client is often aware of the carer's difficulties. What we the carers identified as making us uncomfortable or at a loss with, the clients later identified and were extremely accurate about. This suggests that we should be more honest and address difficulties together with the clients:

'The sister in Casualty who told me my husband was dead was very nice, but she could not cope with it. I had a feeling she would be glad when I left and went home. Several times she said, "You don't want to hang around here, you will be better off at home." Later she said, "Your friends at home will look after you."

I could not take it in. He was a young man, 36 years of age, fit and well. Out jogging and he just dies. I did not want to rush off home. My head was in turmoil. It did not make any sense. I asked her several times if it was true and she became more and more fidgety and distressed. I had seen him dead but thought perhaps it was a nightmare. I wanted to see again if it was true but I knew I was becoming a nuisance.

I suppose it's just in one door, not saved, dead, out of the other door, get the relatives home, ready for the next one. I am not blaming her really but she should have given me more time. I thought afterwards that she probably had a husband the same age as mine. She just could not cope with it.'

This example illustrates how a nurse's difficulty can be apparent to the client. This woman was quite accurate in saying that the sister was in a hurry to get her home. When I interviewed the sister, within 24 hours of the death, she admitted to her difficulty with the woman and her haste to get her off home.

This nurse did indeed have a husband the same age as the client's husband; he too was an avid jogger, and the whole scenario confronted the sister with her own worst fears. If she had been able to recognize this, she could have compensated for it and given the lady more objective and effective care. How we prepare staff to recognize these problems will be explored in Chapter 7 on teaching and training for this type of work.

The nurses in our study identified in relatives nine emotional responses to the news of the sudden death. People experienced and displayed more than one feeling at the same time, although one may have been predominant. Some people experienced opposite ends of the spectrum of emotions, such as acceptance and then denial.

The survey results show the different responses seen in the bereaved person at the time of the death, the number of people in our study expressing them, and the degree of difficulty that nurses had in dealing with them. Note that withdrawal produced the most difficulty and acceptance, crying and sobbing produced the least.

Activity 6A

Which emotional responses do you have the greatest difficulty with? Try to explain why.

Emotional responses to the 100 sudden deaths in descending order of difficulty for the nurses:

- withdrawal   (30)
- denial   (28)
- anger   (27)
- isolation   (24)
- bargaining   (23)
- inappropriate responses   (13)
- guilt   (12)
- crying, sobbing, weeping   (11)
- acceptance   (3)

We will look at each response separately to explore what we mean by it. How the significant relative perceived this response in retrospect will also be discussed. I have found that talking at a later date about how people reacted emotionally on impact is a useful way for them to explore their grief.

WITHDRAWAL

In this state the client becomes inaccessible, mute, and appears to be refusing to listen. This response can leave the carer questioning her effectiveness. In our study and in workshops with other professions involved with the bereaved, the effect of this response on the carer is apparent:

'You wonder if you could have cared for them better.'

'It makes you question the communication skills you have for these situations.'

'You are just left looking at them, feeling helpless.'

If this is explored further with the carer, another difficulty that emerges is the silence. This can be particularly uncomfortable for nurses, whose ethos is about working, caring, or being busy. Nurses have great difficulty in seeing the value of just being there without putting it right. It is not like being able to put a bandage on and 'making it better'. The wound is deep and painful and the attempt at first-aid appears to produce poor results.

Long periods of silence are perceived as sitting doing nothing. The carer searches around for something to do or say. Her efforts appear to fall on deaf ears. The silence is seen by the carer as being of little value, though the client perceives it differently.

The carer feels very vulnerable. This space or time may become a period of self-confrontation as she waits for a response from the client. Several nurses said they started to think what they would do if they were in the client's place. Others described thinking for the first time in a long while about issues such as 'how can God allow this'. Another common thought was how painful and unjust this death was, and how can anyone survive such an experience. To carers in this situation it may seem as if the person does not want them — the client's withdrawal is seen as rejection. Carers then think 'if I have so little to offer, and am so ineffective, perhaps I *should* leave the client alone.' The situation becomes even harder to handle if the carers themselves begin to confront some difficult questions concerning the meaning of life. So it is not hard to understand why there was no hesitation in our group of nurses (and since then in other disciplines) in saying that withdrawal was difficult to tolerate and to understand.

The relatives' perception of withdrawal

'I remember it as if it was yesterday. When they said my son was dead I couldn't speak or move. It struck me down somehow, except I was just sitting there. I remember the nurse. She looked helpless and I thought, "She wants me to do something but what can I do?"

I do not remember how long it lasted but his whole life went before me. Some of it was lovely and made me smile. She (the nurse) looked puzzled as if I was going mad. She got hold of my hand but I was locked into some sort of memory — she's talking about my boy, my son, the first child I gave birth to. I watched him grow, take his first steps. I laughed when he got his words all mixed up.

Dead. What can she mean? This is the boy who was so scared the first day he went to school, but so brave. He could run, run like a hare. How proud he was of his medals. He cannot be dead.

She does not know him. This is my son you are talking about. He was not that clever at school but when he left he was doing all right. That day he brought home his first girl friend. He was shy and embarrassed but tried to be the big, macho man. He was a man, but he cried 6 months later when she left him.

This is my son they are talking about. Dead. "Yes," she said, "the worst has happened. He has died." '

Mrs Brown's withdrawal lasted for 20 minutes as noted on the initial evaluation of her care. This is a long time for a carer to sit in silence whilst someone rocks and smiles to herself occasionally. When we saw Mrs Brown later she did not know about the time lapse. She described how, on impact, she retraced her life with her son, how she tried to make sense of it and how this retracing helped. It brought her back to the present, to the pain and awful impact. She needed this retracing to help her take in what was happening.

Mrs Brown remembered the nurse's discomfort with her withdrawal.

She was not critical of her though, and said, 'I'm so glad she was there with me.' This confirms the value of being able to stay with the pain and distress. It is no easy task, particularly for those who are new to caring for people in this way. When the nurse left the room and she was alone, Mrs Brown was scared. She hoped she would return soon.

There is tremendous value in being able to stay with withdrawal, and our presence is a comfort and strength. We must not assume that no response means rejection and leave the client alone. Unless the client can clearly verbalize that they want to be alone, stay with them.

The retracing that takes place silently in so many people is important. It helps them to understand the death in the context of the whole of their loved one's life. It is the beginning of exploring its meaning, and confronting its pain and disorder. When the client eventually re-emerges from the withdrawal, he or she may begin to tell you about their retracing of steps in the deceased's life. Again this is important in the process of grieving.

To recognize the value of being there, without this being immediately validated, is important for the carer.

DENIAL

Denial of feelings about the death is denial of its reality. In withdrawal, the reality is accepted and work can begin on this. Denial can be clearly expressed as the death not being wanted or acceptable:

'Don't you dare say he is dead.'
'Go away. That cannot be true. I will just go home and forget this.'

Sometimes the fact may be received but the feelings of denial that emerge may surprise even the client: 'How can I be feeling this?' is a common question.

Others comment on the experience being new:

'I have never felt anything like this before. It cannot be true.'
'These feelings are not mine.'
'This is not a part of my life.'
'You must have the wrong person, this is not part of my life scheme or plan. Go away and find the right person.'

The awful imposition of this death on to the person, and the way it interferes with future plans or schemes, is clear here.

If the denial is quickly dissipated it is a relief for the carer. If the denial persists, the carer will question her ability to communicate effectively, is frustrated by this ineffectiveness, and may become more forceful or directive. The carer is left in the invidious position of having to reiterate or reinforce some painful and distressing information.

If someone leaves the scene or hospital in a rigid state of denial we rightly feel anxious about them. This rarely happens, and usually people establish death's awful reality quickly.

Most nurses who give news of sudden death expect denial. They also expect to deal with this and help people to accept death's reality. But if denial persists for 5 minutes or more nurses often become uncomfortable. The person receiving the painful information will ask you to say it is not true. It is difficult and uncomfortable for the bearer of the news to have to confirm pain that is clearly distressing.

There is little wonder then, that denial in relatives rates high as a cause of distress in the carer, when all the carer can do is reinforce the relatives' distress. Nurses see themselves in this act of confirmation as piling on the agony. One nurse described it as being like 'kicking someone when they are down'.

In our study, many of the relatives, evaluated in the immediate situation as displaying marked denial that persisted and was difficult to work with, showed evidence of this in the later visit at 6 or 10 months. Initial denial and difficulty was still present much later. One nurse said:

'I remember Mrs X just would not accept the death of the baby. Her husband and father-in-law colluded with this. When I suggested that she should see and hold the baby they were angry. They were really saying she cannot cope with this, as you can see by the way she is denying it, and still you suggest that.

It was as though I was just adding to her distress, but I felt it was right. She sat and held him, and rocked backwards and forwards, talking to him and then said, "Let's just go home and forget all this. I just want to take my baby home."

I said, "It can't ever be the same, he is dead," and she cried and said, "I know, I just wanted to bury him in the garden so he is near me." Her husband said, "Look what you have done."

When Mrs X was seen later she had left the denial and had begun to grieve about her baby's death. A definite indication from her was that the nurse had helped her a lot. She perceived the immediate struggle with denial as madness.

The struggle for the carer is in helping the client to find acceptable something that is more than just difficult information, to see clearly something that penetrates into their very being. It will frequently make us as carers question what we are doing.

Many people in our study remembered the denial and how they struggled with it, but also how death's awful reality was quickly a part of their existence. It is useful in longer term counselling to recall this immediate struggle and how it was dealt with (or not dealt with) at the time, and to look at how they are working with it now.

ANGER

However short-lived, anger can be frightening; it can push people away from each other leaving them alone and vulnerable. People who are angry lose intellectual clarity and reasoning powers, and are consumed by this powerful emotion.

Anger in grief can cover a wide spectrum: in its mild form people show irritation; at the other extreme they might be in a rage. Irritation is often expressed about some aspect of loss on the periphery, away from the main focus (Fig. 6.1), and may seem inappropriate. In the situation illustrated by the figure, a woman has side-stepped the major focus of her crisis — her husband's death — to some irritating peripheral aspects of her loss. When she returns to the major focus of her crisis she may well experience rage.

Many people label anger as anxiety or fear, because this seems much more acceptable to them and others, including the carer. Anger is often seen as destructive, wicked or sinful; it is rejected or mistrusted, and not seen as the warning device that it is. Anger can be expressed verbally and its cathartic effect produces solutions.

Rage is a much more physical expression of anger and its release is usually damaging. In grief, rage adds to the torment and is a terrifying experience for the carer. For a long time we had a hole in the wall of our relatives' room, as a result of a father's anger at the death of his son in a road traffic accident when someone mentioned that the driver had been going too fast.

Anger directed at the health care system, the doctor or the nurse, can seem much more acceptable than anger directed at the deceased. In my group of nurses, many are prepared for anger being directed at them but are surprised and distressed at its being directed at the deceased.

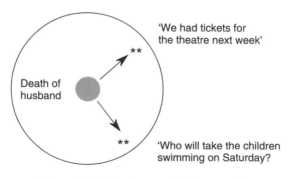

Figure 6.1 Major focus and flight to periphery.

On being told of the death of his son in a motorcycle accident, Mr B said:

'He always was an idiot and now he's gone and got himself killed. You spend all your time working for them, to give them everything, and they do this to you. I will never forgive him for this, never. I hate him.'

When the nurse suggested he did not really mean this and he would see things differently later, he told her to shut up. 'What do you know about it, anyway?' he responded angrily. 'Mind your own business.'

The nurse was very distressed and later described a strong need to defend this person who was unable to defend himself. She also thought his father would regret saying these things, and attempted to put him right.

Carers have a tendency to take responsibility for how people feel, and for those who are unable to defend themselves (in this instance the deceased person). Such issues need clarifying and exploring before undertaking bereavement counselling. We need to be clear about who is responsible for whom, and to realize that this work can become a heavy burden.

Where relatives directed anger towards themselves, carers in our study were able to work with this and usually offer some reassurance, though there were more problems if the deceased had committed suicide.

Our study found that where anger had been a clear response of the client in the immediate situation, it remained a difficulty later on. The focus of the anger may have changed during the 6 or 10 months' interval before follow-up, but it remained a difficulty. If the anger had been directed at the deceased, the relative apologized for this and was embarrassed. One lady who was angry with her husband for working too hard and killing himself as a result of stress, had changed the focus of the anger when seen later:

'I blame his bosses for letting him work like he did. It was only to line their pockets. They reaped all the benefit. Only I was the loser, and him of course. They robbed me of all we had planned for his retirement. That was to be ours and they took it all. I despise the management. I suppose the hate I feel for them is burning me up inside. Just talking about it now could drive me to murder.

If my family knew I was talking like this they would disown me. They say he was a wonderful husband and I should just be thankful for this. Sometimes I think if I had a gun I would have committed murder. I suppose you think I am awful.'

Most people are ashamed of this anger and really value the opportunity of discussing it.

In a counselling relationship, anger is seen as an expression of despair at the loss. Sudden death produces a fight to understand and control the grief of the loss and this can manifest as anger. Carers must be careful not to impose their own feelings about what is appropriate; we all have family rules about anger, how and where it should be expressed.

Anger was in the top three emotional responses producing difficulties for the carer. Many carers, including my nurse group and others from workshops, have expressed fear of being hurt physically when working with sudden death. Few were prepared for this being a possibility.

ISOLATION

Feelings of isolation as expressed by the relatives remind us of our own vulnerability should we be bereaved and left alone. Obviously this is disturbing for the carer but nurses in our study were most uncomfortable with what this meant for the other people (friends or relatives) surrounding the key person. When the key person was given the news of the sudden death or this was confirmed, he or she experienced a sudden sense of isolation or being alone, despite being surrounded by significant and caring people. For example, a common response to the loss of a spouse was:

'I am all alone now.'
'I have nobody.'

If this was followed by another comment about being powerless and helpless, such as:

'All my strength has gone.'
'I have nothing left, nothing to go on for.'

friends and relatives quickly wanted to assure them of their love and support:

'We will be with you.'
'You have all your family and friends.'
'You will not be alone.'

Despite these assurances the bereaved person often continues to express total loss, and feelings of being completely alone and isolated. The distress for the carer appears to stem from the inability of those closest to comfort the bereaved, and from witnessing their distress about this. The carer also feels ineffective when she reminds the bereaved of what is left, because this appears to give little comfort.

Kubler-Ross (1978) describes this sense of isolation, along with denial, as a mechanism of defence until resources can be mobilized, a buffer allowing the client to pull himself together and adopt alternative defences.

In my longer-term counselling, clients have described how, although it distresses friends and relatives, they need people to know that no other person has on offer what the deceased had given them. The powerful and central message at this time is that no one can replace this person or stand in for them, so do not try. When those closest to the bereaved state plainly that they cannot give or have on offer what the deceased did, this becomes less of an issue.

A young woman, whose husband died suddenly at the age of 39 from a heart attack, described how she suddenly felt isolated. She also knew when seen later, that her expression of this had distressed those around her.

'When they said he was dead it was the strangest experience. It was just like being in a big open space, a bit like a desert. It even felt dry and desolate. All these people were around me, my mother and father and brother, and they were all saying we will take care of you. I remember saying, "You cannot, nothing will help me with this."
I was totally alone. There was nothing I or anyone could do. All their words were useless, they were just words. What could they do? I had lost everything. There was nothing left. The more they tried to reassure me the worse it became. I know I just looked, as much as to say "You have nothing for me."
Nothing can comfort or console you when you have lost everything.'

It is not at all unusual for the client to perceive the loss as total. Whatever else they have acquired is of no consolation. Even more painful for those close to them is that they are not seen as a resource. The message they receive is that there is nothing they can offer to help with this. It is difficult for them to be left feeling as helpless as this, and difficult for the carer to witness this predicament.

This most distressing emotional response, reminds us of our inability to put it right. The particular difficulty for doctors and nurses is that in other distressing situations there is often something they can do to offer some comfort. But here you cannot get near the person, they feel totally alone and you are not seen as a resource.

One of the lessons we have to learn in the caring professions is that we cannot always put things right, and that there are some intensely distressing situations where we can only stand by. Eventually, when they are ready, people will begin to emerge from this powerful sense of isolation and will then need some resources. We have somehow to wait on the outside of the pain and be ready to step forward to help and support.

Some people emerge from the feeling of isolation very quickly — that is, within 10 or 15 minutes of impact of death — only to return to this state later. It may be that the impact of the enormity of the loss has to be confronted again before some people can begin to explore other resources. As our group of carers was reminded, this is distressing to witness and leaves us feeling helpless.

BARGAINING

Bargaining in sudden death is where the client attempts to postpone the death by formulating an agreement. He may think that if he alters his behaviour he will prevent the death or be granted an 'extension'. I have witnessed this response most often when the death of a child or young person is involved.

When death is imminent, or news of the death is about to be given and they are aware of what you are about to say, the bargaining begins. This, in my experience, is often about reconciliation with someone they are estranged from, particularly if parents are separated or divorced. There may be remorse for bad behaviour or separation from God. The bargaining may be directed to a specific person or to anyone in the room; some people look heavenward as if appealing to God, whilst others address God by name:

'If you put this right God, I will not let you down again.'
'I will return to the church. I'm sorry, please help me.'

Husbands or wives, or other family members, may appeal to each other:

'From now on we must try to stop arguing and care for our family better. We have failed them. I promise if this can be put right we will all care for each other better.'

Some doctors and nurses are distressed that people will bargain with them for a life:

'I will give you all my money, all I have, if you will save him.'
'No expense must be spared, bring the best people you have. I will find the money somehow. I will sell all I have.'

Despite assurances that the best possible expertise will not save this life, or that the child is already dead, the bargaining may persist. This type of bargaining leaves the carer feeling very uncomfortable, and some are clearly distressed with the idea that money could be an issue in the saving of a life.

Other workers, particularly if they are parents themselves, are distressed at witnessing parents exhorting each other to promise to be good, and having the idea that their bad behaviour has brought this tragedy upon them. In one discussion group, a nurse stated that it reminds you of the frailty and vulnerability of intimate relationships. She did not like the suggestion that the stability of these relationships had an effect on life or death outcomes.

I have counselled several parents who clearly remember bargaining, and I suspect there are many more bargains secretly made with God.

Some people admit to this, but with hindsight feel foolish about it. It is important that with hindsight and after counselling, they usually have a greater sense of our inability to control matters of life and death.

If the counselling has been useful, there will have been a shift from how we control or influence these issues, to what we gain from life each day. Many of the parents I know who have bargained describe it as a desperate attempt to regain control of the situation. They describe a sudden chaos being imposed upon them, and a need to restore order. Alongside this is a desperate need for explanations, for answers to why this is happening.

This need produces a possible explanation — they themselves must have erred from the straight and narrow and their bad behaviour, sin or wickedness has caused this to happen. They then quickly bargain to put it right. Many hours are spent with these people, particularly parents, exploring the meaning of the death and whether it is the outcome of some bad behaviour or sin of theirs.

Some parents actually apologize because they have been selfish in that they were too happy with their children. Others reprimand themselves for never having given a thought to the fact that their child may die, and why should it only happen to others and not theirs. Their search through these issues may be the outcome of their initial bargaining.

When parents are begging forgiveness of each other, with promises to be better in future, this is more distressing. Not only is there an exchange of intimacies that you feel you are intruding upon, but it is difficult to break into and put right. This aspect of bargaining has been the most distressing for the carer in our study.

It would appear that most carers, although experiencing some distress in these situations, are able to respond to them. They can provide reassurance that everything is being done or has been done to save the life, and are able to ask people not to blame themselves and to remind them it was an accident or something they could not have foreseen. Most carers give these assurances quickly, and will therefore be able to offer support and not feel helpless as in some of the previous responses.

INAPPROPRIATE RESPONSES

The emotional response to the news of death can appear inappropriate for the situation, to either the carer or the person receiving the bad news. Lack of response can seem inappropriate. Many suddenly bereaved people are concerned at their immediate numbness and may state:

'Why am I not feeling anything?'
'Should I be going mad now, or breaking down or something?'

In our study, responses seen as inappropriate in the perception of the carer were recorded. Most of the situations recorded involved the responses of an adolescent; something was blurted out which the speaker usually regretted immediately and apologized for, or which produced an angry response from another family member.

John was 15 years old and sat waiting with his father for news of his brother. Simon was 18, and he had only had the motor bike for a month. Now he was lying in the hospital, badly injured. Simon had worked hard to save up for that bike, John thought.

'Will the bike be OK?' John asked his father, when they were both told that Simon might die from his injuries.

'Don't be stupid, John,' his father replied angrily.

Simon wouldn't think it was stupid, John thought, wondering what to say next and not knowing whether to laugh or cry at his father's anger. He often laughed at it lately. He wanted to cry but did not know what to do with his Dad. He had never seen him like this before. He wondered if he should hold his hand, but then thought the nurse might think he was soft.

The doctor came in looking very serious, and began to talk, and his words did not come out properly. How awful, thought John, having a stutter and having to talk to people like this. He half smiled to himself and then saw everyone looking at him disapprovingly.

'I am very sorry, but Simon has just died,' the doctor said to John's father.

John did not know what to do. He felt he had not been told, although he was there. He was desperate to help. My Dad is in such pain, and here am I sitting doing nothing. Please God, tell me what to do, he thought. Give me Simon back. Put it right. After what seemed like an eternity in time, with John looking round the room for something to concentrate on, he said: 'I will have a room of my own now.' With all eyes accusingly on him, he smiled weakly and wished the floor would open and swallow him up.

In our study, people who expressed 'wrong' thoughts or words describe later how uncomfortable, embarrassed and distressed they felt about this. They were often young adolescents struggling to cope with new and difficult feelings. These feelings were powerful and over-whelming, and produced an unfamiliar fear.

The same adolescents describe an intense pressure to help to put things right, of having to respond to reactions in parents that they have never seen or experienced before. More painfully, many adolescents wonder if they are ultimately responsible. In the last case study, John wondered whether it was because 3 days previously, in a discussion with his friend, he had said that God did not exist. A 14-year-old girl whose older sister had died, told me that she had not been doing her homework and had been told that no good would come of it. This tremendous pressure to help and the desperate search for something to take away some of the pain can result in remarks which are unfortunately perceived as inept, stupid or even wicked.

The carer's role is primarily to set a good model through their response to inappropriate remarks, by not being judgmental. We can diffuse some of the anger and difficulty by saying how hard it is to find ways to respond to death, how we are sure they must be at a complete loss as to what to do or say next, and that it is the worst thing in the world for people to find right or proper responses to. Young people need their response and difficulty to be recognized. Adolescents find the crisis situation most difficult — they are neither child or adult; people do not know what to do with them and they do not know what to do with themselves. They should always be included in the breaking of the bad news, in any discussion following it, and in viewing the body.

At the onset of grief everyone's anger is directed at an easy target — a scapegoat. The response that seems inappropriate may act as a trigger for the mechanism of 'scapegoating' to occur. For example, John could easily have been the target of everyone's anger. He and his family needed help to cope with and understand his feelings and ambivalence in order to avoid this.

GUILT

Remorse, the feeling that we are in some way to blame for the sudden death, is very common. The most frequent expression of this is guilt at failing to act or respond usefully or effectively:

'I was too slow in calling the ambulance.'
'I should have made him see a doctor.'
'I didn't want to travel on the route on which he was killed.'
'I should have made him wait to drive. He was too tired.'

It may be that because the person is not there to take responsibility for himself, we have to take it for him. For some, it is disrespectful or culturally unacceptable to make negative remarks about dead people. This attitude will not only produce problems in the immediate situation, but also in the later stages of grieving.

The death is often felt to be a punishment. The client is left with a feeling that he has behaved in a way that is inconsistent with his internal value system or conscience. Some will say that they have sinned against God and that this is the outcome. A voice inside them states that their behaviour needs correcting and that this death is the sign that confronts them with that. The sudden death, as the outcome or punishment, is the ultimate message or reminder of having done something wrong by commission or omission.

Guilt is not always inappropriate, and carers describe this as being especially difficult. When a drunken driver kills a spouse or a friend, it is appropriate that they should feel bad about it. If a drunken driver kills himself, people feel guilty about being angry with him for being so stupid. It is very easy to feel guilty.

Many situations evoke feelings of guilt and present a challenge to work with, for example ill health, sexual activity, surviving an accident when others have died. Helping the client to learn to forgive himself or others, and move forward, is required. Whilst some guilt is appropriate, some is excessive for the situation, and unhealthy. Help from carers to cope with this at immediate impact can affect how people struggle with the guilt later.

The difficulties of being the survivor of a sudden death, particularly an accident, may result in feelings of shame:

'I could have saved him.'
'It should have been me that died.'

If someone is found out and exposed, or if, in the review of the events, a person feels to blame, he is left with shame. I heard a disaster worker say that, in working with survivors, she had never encountered so much shame. Shame is about exposure to self and others, and about being looked at or having fingers pointed at you. Blame and its resulting shame may stem from being found out or the threat of being found out. Shame reflects the character of the person, and has consequences.

The other problem about guilt, in the immediate or long term, is that it may be the result of parental programming. Parental messages of 'should' and 'ought' act as a conscience, and a person may be left believing that when anything goes wrong they are to blame. What could be more wrong than a sudden death? In the immediate situation, the difficulty for carers is that they wonder where to begin with this powerful programming.

In the immediate situation of sudden deaths in our study, nurses perceived that guilt became an issue in the majority of cases. It was certainly an issue for most clients in the long term. A question worth asking was: is that why they responded to our request for help in our study? Did it offer some way of making amends, or offer some help in the search to minimize the guilt?

The search to understand the reason for a death quickly leads on to issues related to guilt, to how much control we have over our lives, and whether this is governed by good and evil. For some, issues of good and evil are perfectly clear. If somebody's sudden death is the result of a crime it may be seen clearly as being due to evil, sin and wickedness. It is very difficult for people to say:

'It was an accident, he was in the wrong place at the wrong time, we could not foresee this.'

We seem to have a need to feel that we control our destiny and have complete authority over what happens to us. The fact that we do not have this power can make us feel uneasy, uncomfortable or out of control.

One difficulty in dealing with a client's guilt is the very private nature of it. Whilst they may reveal some of it, there is often a discomfort at having done so, and a reluctance to proceed further. Carers are naturally uncomfortable with this, as further questioning may make us and the client aware of guilt's oppressive nature and its shame.

If the guilt response is excessive, we may attempt to reduce its impact, but if the guilt appears wholly appropriate in our perception of the event, we may be reluctant to try to take it from the client or lessen its impact.

A common response from the carer (nurses in our study) about guilt on impact was the enormity of the problem. Many felt, quite rightly, that there were so many other immediate tasks that we could have some influence on and work effectively with, that guilt would have to remain a long-term issue for the client to work with. Despite this, we should address sensitively the issues linked with guilt, and not avoid them at immediate impact. I often suggest the feeling is wholly appropriate, by saying something like:

'That will be something you will need to think about, and perhaps talk to someone about.'

We should not dismiss as wholly inappropriate guilt issues that appear to be excessive for the situation. They are a valid difficulty for the client, who must not be made to feel stupid about them. Failure to work with the guilt may prevent someone working through the grief process:

'You read so much these days about fats and cholesterols and how we should avoid them. I had read it all, and just ignored it. My husband was only young really. Well, 41 years is not old. He played football and was doing so when he died. He smoked and liked his beer, and he loved that fatty bit on the joint of meat. We used to kid him on about it, and say it will be the death of you yet, but never once believing it would.

The death certificate said something about fat in his arteries. I know it's stupid but I never did anything to prevent that. We just pay lip service to so much, but we do nothing about it. The morning he died I gave him a big, fatty bacon sandwich. He loved them.

The thought of it now makes me sick. Since reading that death certificate I have not bought any bacon. I avoid it like the plague in the supermarket. When the lads asked why we didn't have any, I went crackers and started shouting at them. They couldn't understand it.

That sandwich tipped the balance. It took him over the edge. It killed him in the end, and I gave him it.'

There are situations where issues of blame and guilt, and who carries it, will prevent the grief process taking place. After these issues have been publicly discussed at inquests, there can be further progress in the grieving or an even firmer stance on blame and guilt. Legal wrangling over compensation, and putting a monetary value on someone's life and death, can further complicate matters.

CRYING, SOBBING AND WEEPING

Catharsis, or the release of strong feelings, has long been considered an important component of the therapeutic process. Freud (1910) discovered that no lasting benefit was produced by an outpouring of feelings, but that the release reduced anxiety and depression. Freud also observed that weeping motivated the client to remain in therapy. In my longer-term counselling of bereaved clients, I find they often feel they have achieved something if there is an overt outpouring of grief in the session. It is not always clear what constitutes emotional arousal. A short burst of crying, quickly controlled, may signify intense arousal in a shy, inhibited individual.

Crying, sobbing and weeping will produce very different responses from observers, depending on the culture and sex of the person expressing the feeling. In a Western culture people are often more comfortable with this response in a woman. People continue to be embarrassed when men cry, and in particular men themselves if the others present are women. Some Asian groups of men will cry openly and comfortably together without women being present.

A common response to sudden death is crying, sobbing and weeping, and most people, including the person crying, have a sense of its appropriateness. Sadness or grief, when expressed as crying or sobbing, is often felt to be a good thing, and people wait for it to happen. It is perceived as a release of pain and distress. Most of the anxiety about it concerns when it will stop. Many express a fear of its being unending, and draining away energy. When it happens you could say the person is suffering, and yet it is greatly valued by both lay and professional people.

Control is a word often used in relation to expression of sorrow. Losing control of one's feelings, or the inability to keep them internalized, verges on madness for some people. Loss of emotional control can easily be equated with insanity.

Most people, when seen later in our study, felt they had no difficulty with this response to the impact. They felt it made it easier for people to care for and comfort them. Of all the emotional responses to sudden death, crying was seen in the most positive light. More people speak of the value of this than of any other response discussed. Also, crying, sobbing and weeping facilitated physical contact more than any other response.

This response also produced the least difficulty for the nurses in my study. It appealed to their need to feel useful, and gave them something to do in physically comforting weeping people. Crying was easily understood as a response to sudden death, and felt to be wholly appropriate and somehow more manageable.

A study by Brewis (1989) of police officers, and how they react to dealing with sudden death, showed the opposite response. Police officers were less able to cope with crying, sobbing and weeping, and found withdrawal easier to tolerate. This was felt to be due to their role and conditioning. Police officers are taught to apply the law and not allow emotional considerations to impair their judgement. This emotional distancing from the client takes place many times in their daily work. So withdrawal, and the distancing this produces, is tolerated more easily than crying which evokes a nurturing response that they are less comfortable with than the nurses. This difference in how the person in the carer's role reacts has implications in identifying training needs. Brewis' study, which concerns informing relatives about a sudden death, found that policemen experienced greater stress on receiving the call to visit the house than with breaking the bad news.

The only difficulty with crying, described by two or three young female nurses in our study, was at witnessing men cry. They went on to say that it confronted them with the fact that their own fathers were vulnerable and could cry; they did not want to be reminded of this.

It is important to note here that people do not always want physical contact or to be comforted; we must be prepared to be rejected.

ACCEPTANCE

Acceptance is a term used in grief work to describe the final stage of grieving, when the client has had sufficient time to work through the previous stages. Acceptance occurs when most of the emotional pain has gone and the struggle with the loss is over.

It is a difficult surprise to some carers that, on hearing the news of a sudden death, a few people appear to accept and not struggle with this information. They are not in a state of denial, and their perception is not altered or impaired; they simply receive and accept the loss. Although distressed, they may give feedback to show they have heard and are in touch with its reality.

Sometimes a previous loss has prepared such people for this one. The experience is not new and this can make the present impact less powerful.

Some people will have discussed the possibility of sudden death with the deceased and have made contingency plans for it. They know that sudden death is possible in all our lives, and not only will they not have denied or avoided this, but will have had open discussion of it with loved ones. Others will have validated their love for each other before the event, along with the acknowledgement of death being a possibility, and will therefore have no unfinished business, nothing left unsaid or undone. This situation may be difficult for an outsider to accept, but some people do use opportunities to the full, and will feel, even in crisis, a sense of having completed something.

Because we usually see sudden death resulting in disorder, we may have difficulty with or feel uncomfortable about acceptance of the death on impact. Our experience of acceptance is that it is the final stage of grief, and because of this, most carers involved in the impact of the sudden death will want to check that the client is not in a state of denial. Many carers will remain uncomfortable if someone has been able to receive and quickly work with the impact of sudden death; we must remember that this is our problem, not theirs.

In this chapter we have looked at emotional responses in relatives on impact of sudden death. We have not only identified what the carer has difficulty in responding to at this time, but also what problems, with hindsight, the client experienced in his own responses. In gaining some insight into what clients experienced with these emotional responses, and how they perceived the carer's response, we begin to clarify some of the skills required for this work.

REFERENCES

Brewis T 1989 Stress and reactions of police officers when warning relatives of a sudden or unexpected death. Unpublished study for West Yorkshire Police for HND
Copp L A 1993 Treatment, torture, suffering and compassion. Journal of Professional Nursing 6(1):1–2
Freud S 1910 Two short accounts of psycho-analysis. Reprinted 1966. Penguin, Harmondsworth
Kubler-Ross E 1978 To live until we say goodbye. Prentice Hall, NJ, USA

7

Teaching and training to care

This chapter examines some of the stated needs of people working with sudden death. It examines concepts to be formally taught and describes workshop games and exercises that focus on particular issues of communication and skill. The exercises used are well tried and tested, and evaluated by hundreds of participants as being useful in such trainings.

During the past 5 years, one third of my time has been taken in teaching and training people of many disciplines to work with sudden death. The amount of time personnel are allowed 'out of work' to focus on this subject has diminished. Many of my training sessions are for one day only and organizations have increased the number of personnel attending each time. Smaller groups of 12–15, over 2–3 days, would be more effective and valued and provide a safer environment. In general, the workshops provide an informal and relaxed way of teaching a difficult subject. The suggestions which follow here are not set out in any particular order, but offered to be used in training sessions as appropriate. There is a recent shift towards self-directed learning, allowing some control over the pace and input. However, the nature of the subject and the feelings that are aroused, mean that people should always have quick access to course leaders and tutors. Some sources for self-directed learning are given in the reference list.

Some people have expressed anxiety about the distress experienced by some participants on my courses, and worry about what distress people might take away. My argument is that those who work in caring for the suddenly bereaved need to know about their own vulnerability. It is better to discover it in the training session than to be overwhelmed by it when with the clients. Our vulnerability must not prevent us from caring effectively for clients. Any unresolved difficulties need to be confronted. After training sessions, some will know they are not yet ready to do this sort of work. The trainer should be able to advise where they can go for further help.

Clients' attitudes and responses to sudden death are diverse, and even if different from our own or from what we may have witnessed previously, they are equally valid. There is no right or wrong response to sudden death, and this is the subject of many discussions in training sessions. In training for and exploring responses of clients and ourselves, we are not concerned about the right or wrong of responses, but about the nature of these responses. We are not dealing with aberrations or clinical signs of 'illness' but human responses to an overwhelming difficulty — sudden death.

The training is intended to help us to help clients more effectively. That may mean doing nothing, or simply helping them to make use of available resources. Some of the difficult encounters in crisis intervention, and how much power or control the carer can have in each situation, can be usefully explored before the event in workshops. This enables carers to be more personally and professionally effective, when the nature of the work could easily have the opposite effect and leave us feeling burnt out.

The aim of our training sessions is to arm carers with insights and responses to the difficulties they will encounter. It is important to give carers permission to examine their own needs as well as those of the clients. Carers often find this difficult; it can feel rather self-indulgent. Although we hope to help the carer return to a position of strength, this need not conflict with the need to focus on and identify vulnerability.

The presence of carers at a training session is a sign of their commitment to working with the very difficult situation of sudden death. Many will have a lot of experience in this, and their presence is a chance for them to re-evaluate what they know, and to share it. It is often difficult in the work setting to look objectively at what we do and the knowledge we have acquired; the training session helps us do that. This chapter is intended to encourage carers to take part in such workshops, and also to provide guidelines for those considering running training sessions.

POSITIVE AND NEGATIVE EXPERIENCES OF CARE WORKERS

For this exercise, workshop participants are asked to produce a list of all that they bring into crisis situations that is positive, and then a list of what they feel is negative. When a composite list is compiled on a board at the front of the room, it will be apparent that some things can be put on both lists. An example of this might be 'persistent encounters with death'.

BRAINSTORMING NEEDS OF CARE WORKERS

The need for a structure to work with in crisis intervention can be examined in a brainstorming exercise. People are asked to identify their needs or what will help to equip them for the work. This also highlights expectations of themselves or of the day's training. Some of the needs quickly identified at the start of our training days are as follows:

- interpersonal skills
- help with words to communicate sensitively
- help with feelings and attitudes of the bereaved
- insights into responses
- structured ways of working
- response to difficult behaviour such as anger or high activity
- to be able to handle the stress.

Covering these key issues may need several sessions. The exercise can also highlight deficiencies within an organization. This can be explored further by discussing, in small groups, what we as carers should take some personal responsibility for. There are likely to be some very different views on this.

Another way of looking at organization difficulties is as follows. One group is 'given' unlimited resources of people and money and asked to use this to set up good support structures for helping carers remain effective in the work of caring for the suddenly bereaved. Another group works with very limited resources and must use them effectively and prioritize needs. The outcomes from both groups are then compared.

WHAT IS COPING?

In very simple terms, coping concerns our response to change. Lazarus (1966), in his studies of coping behaviour, described two ways of coping with a situation that we find stressful and which has the potential for crisis. We can change the stressful situation itself, perhaps by altering our responses or feelings about it. Alternatively, we can manage the stress rather than altering it, by direct action or by avoidance. Some typical and common diversions from stress are smoking, drinking, taking drugs and overeating. These can make stress more tolerable by avoidance, and are one way of managing it.

A workshop exercise could ask two groups to look at these two ways of coping and to give examples from their own encounters with the stress of sudden death. The exercise highlights how a person handles demands and conflicts from within and without, and identifies how we tolerate or minimize these. Coping includes the way we handle the feelings, thoughts and bodily responses of others. There is no one way of coping with a situation. How we cope will depend on our past experience, personality, relationship with others and our environment. We need to look at all of these dimensions when considering coping.

How the carer sees the client as coping with sudden death may be examined in another exercise for two groups. One group is asked to write 10 statements on 'Coping is...' and the other on 'Coping is not...'. Certain items may appear on both lists, and this can provide some amusement. A common example is: 'Coping is not crying' and 'Coping is crying.'

A third exercise on coping is to discuss the following statement about a bereaved client after a sudden death:

'What did you want the client to take away?'

This can be an exercise for two groups, one adding to the statement 'in the immediate care,' and the other 'after long-term counselling'. This exercise looks at the expectations and goals of counselling, and will highlight our assumptions about change or about allowing the client to be themselves with the carer in a comforting or nurturing role. Are the desired outcomes for us or for the client? For example, the carer might be rejected as having nothing to offer the client. How will we respond to this? Does anyone in the helping role consider this response as a possibility?

DEALING WITH EMOTIONAL RESPONSES

The previous chapter identified some of the emotional responses we are confronted with in sudden death. The nature of each of these responses and the difficulties we have in dealing with them can also be explored in workshops. Knowledge of the various theories on loss and the processes of grief is valuable. Carers also need an ability to stay with the pain, anguish and distress of the sufferer, as this validates where clients are and how they feel. Exploring some of the responses described in the previous chapter enables us to stay with our feelings and those of our clients and have some insight into the human response to grief.

Where the various responses fit in to the overall processes of grief, and the care of the client, is also important. The impact of the sudden death is overwhelming and sometimes chaotic. The disorder it produces for us and for our clients can make it unmanageable. Carers need to manage both the disorder and themselves. This immediate management affects the immediate or long-term coping strategies of clients.

Using holistic care in the process of coping with crisis requires a knowledge both of theories and their practical application. The skills involved are not magic solutions, but offer ways to make the situation more manageable and to understand the disordered behaviour. Staff working with sudden death will need some formal teaching of these theories (see Chapter 1) and their application to practice. The usefulness of working models, or the constraints these structures impose upon the care worker, can be discussed in small groups. The exercise of fitting clients into the model or process of working usually produces lively discussion.

INTERPERSONAL SKILLS FOR DIFFICULT SUBJECTS

Working with a client's life crisis requires some good interpersonal skills, as discussed earlier regarding breaking the bad news. We can practise these skills through exercises on listening, establishing eye contact and finding the right words. It can be surprisingly challenging to hear ourselves say out loud words such as dying and dead, for example. Often carers avoid pain or distress by saying things like 'We have lost her' or 'He has slipped away.' The words in the following list can be said out loud to another person in a pairs exercise.

Loss	Death	Coffin
Dead	Divorce	Mourning
Dying	Custody	Grave
Gone	Abandoned	Cremated
Absent	Grieving	Buried
Bereft		

As person A says the words out loud to person B, B attempts to pick up any difficulties the speaker has from inflections in the voice or from hesitations. A is asked, whilst saying them, to try to be aware of which words cause him difficulty or painful memories. Then, without discussion, the roles are immediately reversed with B saying the words out loud to A. The difficulties, or pain, or reluctance to use certain words, are then discussed together.

When debriefing this exercise in open discussion, issues will be raised about the rituals of death and the confrontational nature of the words. Note that the words in the third column of the list are all related to ritualistic responses to death.

Other words, such as custody, divorce and separation offer a stimulus to discuss the differences, if any, between these issues and death. This discussion should highlight the major loss experienced in the former transactions, and how they may stigmatize or embarrass even more than death does. They are certainly subjects people avoid as much as death. Many people describe the anger and distress they feel when the grief of divorce is not recognized and is avoided as much as death.

The exercise just discussed requires some trust, an openness and an honesty between the people sharing the exercise. These qualities can be related to the key words we already have for learning and working with clients:

- trust
- openness
- honesty
- sharing.

The difficulty of establishing these qualities, and others that may occur, can be usefully discussed near the end of a study day. This helps to identify the many-faceted qualities needed for good interpersonal skills.

PERSONAL EXPERIENCE OF DEATH

The material you collect from your own personal experience within your family and culture can be either a hindrance or an asset. If death and its pain were denied, hidden away and not openly discussed, you may have problems working with it. You may have remained in this state of denial. Alternatively you may have compensated so much for this, that you are too direct about death and this may be perceived by some clients as being insensitive and confronting.

It is essential, therefore, that we know ourselves, understand something of the nature of our family's response to death, and acknowledge something of our cultural backgrounds. Our personal characteristics and life experiences must be examined, otherwise we will have problems if these re-emerge in a disruptive or painful way with the client.

In my workshops people often apologize because they have no personal experience of sudden death, or any death for that matter, in their own families. Others sometimes suggest that it is the ultimate qualification to do the work. A lively discussion ensues if you make the statement:

'You only really know the pain and impact of death if you have experienced it yourself.'

It obviously produces some anxiety to take part in an exercise that examines our own experiences of death. As well as examining the issues involved in our 'whole life' encounter with death, it is valuable to look at the difficulties of doing such an exercise. This will reflect communication issues experienced daily by our clients, and highlights how vulnerable they feel when sharing such difficulties.

One way of looking at our own life experience and exploring its impact on us, is to use a questionnaire (Fig. 7.1). Wordon (1983) compiled the series of questions in Fig. 7.1 to help carers look at their own losses. He pointed out that the type of client the carer will have personal difficulty with is usually related to the carer's own area of unresolved conflict.

I have collected 500 such questionnaires, completed by people who work with sudden death — nurses, doctors, social workers, counsellors from many fields of work, voluntary workers, residential care staff and

1. The first death I can remember was the death of:	
2. I was aged:	
3. The feelings I remember I had at the time were:	
4. The first funeral (wake or other ritual service) I ever attended was for:	
5. I was aged:	
6. The thing I most remember about that experience is:	
7. My most recent loss by death was:	
(person, time, circumstances)	
8. I coped with this loss by:	
9. The most difficult death for me was the death of:	
10. It was difficult because:	
11. Of the most important people in my life who are now living, the most difficult death for me would be the death of:	
12. It would be the most difficult because:	
13. My primary style of coping with loss is:	
14. I know my grief is resolved when:	
15. It is appropriate for me to share my own experience of grief with a client when:	

Figure 7.1 Questionnaire — Personal experience of death. (Reprinted from Wordon 1983 with permission.)

policemen. They have given me a wealth of information. In workshop settings, I usually give people 15–20 minutes to fill in the questionnaire. As it is a very confronting exercise it may be best done at the end of the morning session, before a break.

The questions cover our life's history of confrontations with death, from childhood, to our fears for the future and our ideas on coping. The facilitator should remain present whilst the form is being completed, as some people will need questions clarified and others may find feelings of grief re-emerge. Most people find the exercise useful in encouraging work they have not done for themselves on grief.

Whilst the exercise is useful on a personal level, the 500 forms provide a lot of useful general information about what happens to people as they encounter death, both in their family and as individuals. They may also provide some insight as to why these people in particular have chosen to help others with sudden death.

The questionnaire can be broken up into sections when discussing it later, to examine issues linked with each group of questions in turn. People could be asked to pair up with someone (preferably a person they have carried out one previous short exercise with but who is otherwise a stranger) and then asked to discuss for 10 minutes with each other: 'Any issue that you were confronted with by the questionnaire.' The facilitator should note any difficulties encountered by participants. Below are some behavioural signs indicating difficulty:

- a reluctance to begin the exercise
- a quick completion of the exercise, avoiding eye contact or intimacy with the partner
- physical closeness may be apparent, and making physical contact; giving each other good attention
- being embarrassed at obvious distress, or responding to it comfortably
- looking around the room uncomfortably, observing whether others are able to take part in the exercise
- tight-lipped and rigid demeanour, throwing hostile glances towards the facilitator; resentment at the exercise is apparent
- when told it is time to stop, how long does it take them to disengage from the interaction?

Some of the above observations may be made known to the group after they have discussed the exercise together. In debriefing the exercise, a list is made of the difficulties participants encountered in the 10-minute interaction and with the questionnaire. Some difficulties commonly listed are as follows:

- makes you feel vulnerable
- unresolved loss re-emerges
- difficulty controlling emotions
- resentment/anger at being asked to reveal personal material
- finding the right words
- time constraint
- lack of privacy
- is it easier with a stranger?

This exercise reminds us that, in our interactions with clients, the clients experience all these difficulties. This is what it feels like to be asked to share feelings of grief and loss. We can become blasé and insensitive about inviting people to share pain and distress; it is, in fact, an awkward thing to do. We should not forget how embarrassed and vulnerable the client can feel when sharing pain and distress.

Another issue for discussion concerns the conditions or surroundings we offer people to talk in. Lack of privacy, feelings emerging where others are present or overhearing, may also be considered in debriefing this exercise. Many hospitals are poor at providing areas where people can hear bad news with privacy. Distressed people have been told of someone's sudden death in a corridor where they were overheard, or where many people were passing. Others described sitting in an office where people interrupted to answer telephones or collect materials.

The personal questionnaire exercise highlights how it feels to share sensitive things in public or exposed surroundings. The value of providing private rooms and facilities for the suddenly bereaved needs more attention. Clients may later become fixed on difficulties linked with this.

Looking at the questionnaire in more detail

I have now used this exercise at least a hundred times, and in the evaluation of courses and study days have noted the ambivalence of the participants. Most care workers value the exercise but are very much aware of its personal impact. Many are surprised at the strength of feeling that re-emerges. Most need a little time to experience the subject before it is developed further, and to get in touch with some of their feelings.

If I have only one day, I prefer to use the exercise somewhere in the middle of the day, so that participants have time to recover from some of its impact before they leave. It is worth advising them before beginning that it would not be unusual if some people were distressed by the exercise.

The questionnaire usually produces some lively discussions, and particular issues can be linked with the different questions. Participants are surprisingly willing to share personal encounters with death, and this will highlight differences in experience and how the differences are perceived. Some people will feel that their family's experience of and response to death was healthy and useful; others will say the opposite.

Questions 1–6 (see Fig. 7.1) usually bring up issues about children, childhood and family responses to death and community responses.

Discussion about the age at which children understand about the concept of death and its meaning produces many anecdotes. A common source of anger and resentment, and one apparent in my questionnaires, concerns being excluded from a grandparent's funeral as a child. Many describe returning home from school to discover relatives in the house and the funeral over. Others learnt of the death from a person other than a parent, and are angry that parents were unable or failed to tell them.

This discussion may lead on to the community's response to death. Older people will describe relatives lying in a coffin in the 'front room' and the ritual drawing of the curtains. All the neighbours, and the community, could see the clear signs of a death. Others will describe how, nowadays, there are few signs of death and people discover a neighbour has died many weeks after the event.

Questions 7–10 look at recent personal encounters with death and can be used to examine some of the stresses of working with sudden death. It is useful to consider the difficulty of separating our own losses from our work by posing a problem such as 'How do you work with the death of someone's mother or father, when you have just experienced the death of your own?'

Discussion on separating our own grief from the client's, and focusing on our own needs, is usually animated. I am constantly reminded in these discussions how carers ask for very little for themselves. Somehow it is seen as self-indulgence, and the carer's expectations of themselves are often outrageous. We do not demand from our clients what we demand from ourselves. Someone will always describe going back to work after the statutory 3 days compassionate leave, and expecting themselves, or being expected to, become re-immersed in caring for the bereaved immediately. Anxiety is always expressed that to state this is difficult, or to ask for help is a sign of weakness, or that it will be recorded against them.

Another problem is that there are often few or no resources within the system to care for or counsel the staff. When I begin to discuss the needs and difficulties stemming from the staff's personal encounters with death, they often become quiet. Why is it difficult for them to talk about their own needs? Does it say something about the carers, that with other people's difficulties they feel needed or powerful or in a position of strength, but are unwilling to deal with their own needs?

Discussion of the personality profiles of carers rarely fails to provoke interesting responses.

Half the people filling in the questionnaire will fail to answer questions 11 and 12 honestly. Many will refuse to answer them and simply put a line through them. Others will have put someone's name down and crossed it out. Trying to be honest in answering these two questions produces guilt and conflict. Very few are comfortable with and clear about their answer.

Question 11 asks you to name *one* person and few are able to do this. Those who are mothers of more than one child will say it is impossible to say one child's loss would be more difficult than another's. I would refute that. Many parents whom I have seen for long-term counselling have needed to discuss difficulties with their grief, because one child's death is commonly more difficult than another's; our relationships with each of our children are unique and valued for different reasons. Likewise, in the case of adults, one person's death may well be more difficult than another's. Some participants will reject this question because they do not want to explore it. However, if we are going to work with sudden death at its onset or later, we must be aware of our *own* worst fears.

When we are confronted with these fears in others, and particularly if we have to work with them, we need to understand why the work can be especially difficult. When we are confronted with our own worst fears in our clients, we are likely to be less effective and consequently to struggle with the work. The difficulty will be worse if we deny the connection with being confronted with our own worst fears. If we acknowledge this difficulty we will find some way of compensating for it. More than that, we will forgive ourselves for finding the interaction difficult. We will then have some insight into how our fears can make us less effective.

In an earlier case study (see Chapter 6), where a nurse rushed a bereaved woman out before she was ready to go back home, the nurse had been confronted with her own worst fears and refused to acknowledge this. The client was clearly aware of the nurse's difficulty, and later remarked on it:

'She must have had a husband the same age as mine. She could not cope with me.'

Question 12 need not be pursued in the workshop setting. The issues around it are acknowledged in Question 11, and can remain with the individual.

Questions 13 and 14 can be used for a short discussion on how our views on coping vary. Another exercise, What is coping?, was described earlier in this chapter. The word 'resolved' in Question 14 deserves particular attention. It highlights issues of grief, and discussion on whether resolution is too high an expectation. The question arises: Is grief ever resolved? This is an example of how one word can produce much teaching material from the group.

Finally, Question 15 illustrates how the experience of grief is a unique and individual one. It is easy to dilute someone else's experience or distract or divert them from it to your own. That may suit us if we are having difficulty with the client's pain. How can you make use of your own experience in a constructive and sensible way?

One suggested rule about this is to offer your own material only if asked to. I have rarely been asked at the impact of loss, and would certainly not offer it at this time. In long-term counselling, however, clients often need a glimpse of the person behind the role of counsellor. They often ask the counsellor to reveal vulnerability about themselves. In this situation it seems more appropriate.

The exercise using this questionnaire will require at least $1^1/_2$ hours in total. The deaths we have experienced fit into a whole life experience — from childhood to present losses and on to fears of future losses. It is helpful to end by discussing how we feel about coping with all this. The exercise is difficult, and people can be congratulated for taking part and encountering a sometimes painful glimpse of themselves. It is also important to be reminded of how we expect clients to do this.

> **Activity 7A**
>
> Discuss why a participant in this exercise may feel angry about being asked to do it.

It is not at all unusual for unresolved difficulties to emerge from this exercise, and if people are to be effective in this work the difficulties may require further time and attention. Participants may need to talk further with a friend or colleague. Many of the questions offer the care worker a chance to examine personal difficulties. This exercise is essential for people involved in long-term bereavement counselling.

SHARING FEELINGS ABOUT LOSS

How we feel and behave when we discover the loss of something we value reflects some of the overall difficulties experienced in sudden death. An exercise that looks at this but also encourages course participants to meet and talk to each other is the 'Searching' game.

Participants are asked to pair up with someone in the room whom they do not know. After a few minutes spent introducing themselves to each other they begin the exercise, sitting facing each other so they can give each other full attention. They are asked to spend 3 minutes each describing how they felt on discovering the loss of some object that they have valued; it must not be a person or a living thing such as a pet. It may help to remember an incident where something was borrowed and never returned, or stolen, or lost through carelessness. As well as noting how they felt on discovering the loss, they are asked to say how they set about finding the object. The person listening is asked to help her partner share his feelings about the loss.

After both partners have had their turn, the group is asked to contribute to two lists on a board: one headed 'feelings', and the other 'behaviour'. The list headed 'feelings' concerns how they felt on discovering the loss. Below is a typical response:

- anger directed at self
- anger directed at others
- denial
- sadness
- panic
- regret
- acceptance
- resignation
- confusion
- fear
- anxiety

- resentment
- suspicion
- hope.

These words will help to stimulate discussion.

The 'behaviour' list shows how they set about finding the object. Some typical responses are:

- panic/disorder/chaos
- searching — disordered
  — more orderly
- retracing steps
- compulsive/obsessive behaviour
- concealment
- intense activity
- inactivity (resignation)
- enlisting help
- replacing
- diversions
- defensive (bolts, padlocks etc.).

Again, the words on the list provide a stimulus to discussion. The two lists give participants a glimpse of themselves and their responses to losses.

Participants can go on to explore which feelings and behaviours they are more accepting of within themselves or others, and which they become angry about or find unacceptable. This helps to identify feelings and responses we have an inbuilt difficulty with.

Finally, the lists can be used to help participants think about responses to sudden death by identifying those on the list that have arisen with suddenly bereaved people they have met. Some of these responses a carer will find more manageable, others will be very distressing and difficult to respond to. It will become apparent as you explore the responses further that intense, disordered or chaotic behaviour is most difficult for the carer, the client, his family and friends to tolerate. Feelings, although painful, somehow seem easier for the carer to respond to. Certain behaviours will add to the sense of disorder, loss of control, and potential for madness. It is no wonder that carers have problems coping with this on personal, professional and skills levels.

This exercise can take 1–2 hours.

EXPERIENCING SILENCE

Silence in the immediately bereaved was identified in the previous chapter as something that makes carers feel uncomfortable. This exercise shows us how to stay with and identify feelings without verbalizing them. It is carried out in pairs, each person taking some stance that describes a feeling, e.g. withdrawal, agitation, perplexity. Participants are asked to think of feelings on discovering a loss as identified in the previous exercise.

Person A acts out non-verbally the feeling and B mirrors this. B should make every effort to mirror A exactly, taking particular note of the position of the head, limbs, feet and distribution of weight. After A has spent 5 minutes initiating the non-verbalized feelings, it is then B's turn.

The exercise ends with discussion of how participants felt about their closeness to the other person's feelings. Which feeling could they emulate most easily and relate most to, and which left them feeling uncomfortable?

Another exercise to examine the difficulty of silence is to spend 2 minutes in three different postures, in silence:

1. back to back
2. side by side
3. facing each other with knees touching.

Participants then discuss what they learnt about themselves and others by doing this.

Whilst the exercises concerning silences have much to teach us, they can also be fun. This is a necessary ingredient in a day dealing with sudden death.

REFLECTING FEELINGS

We have already identified that it is easier to work with the feelings behind the behaviour in crisis intervention. Difficult and disordered behaviour causes distress for the carer as well as for the client. The shift to the feelings underlying the behaviour helps to put some order and meaning into the situation, and explains some of the disorder.

This next exercise helps with focusing on feelings and practising putting them into words. Participants are split up into pairs and A talks to B for 4 minutes about an incident which produced a lot of feelings. This could be something from childhood, or a holiday incident which perhaps produced anxiety as well as pleasure. B then reflects the feelings but not the content, for 2 minutes. Partners then swop over.

When working with sudden death it helps us if we can evaluate where the client is in his grieving process. In this situation, we need to allow ourselves to be wrong, to have used the wrong word to describe how they are feeling and to be able to say:

'I see, do you mean...'

and then offer another word. The following exercise gives practice in identifying and describing feelings. It provides another way of gaining a wider vocabulary of feelings which will help us to describe the client's feelings.

To begin, draw a line down the middle of a sheet of paper and write two words that describe opposite extremes of feeling (e.g. happy to sad, Fig. 7.2), one at the top and the other at the bottom. Then write down words in between that describe feelings along this spectrum. After spending 5 minutes on this, work in small groups to share the difficulties and the words you find useful or apt for situations. Participants can then discuss how some words describe such extreme distress and are so powerful that we are reluctant to use them. Try other ranges of feelings, for example irritation to rage.

The wider vocabulary to describe feelings gained from the above exercise should help us become more sensitive to the level of feeling that clients have reached in their grief process.

A variation on this exercise is to look at the line and the words at the top and bottom. Begin in the middle by describing a situation and take it

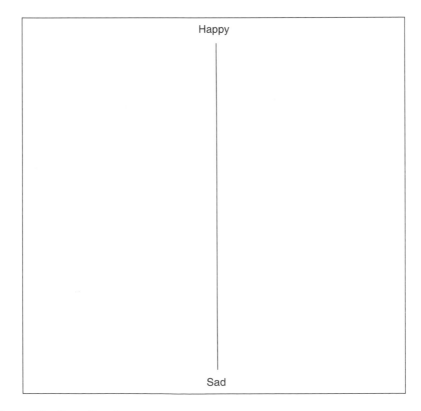

Figure 7.2   Opposite extremes.

to an extreme. This should highlight how people often begin somewhere safe and how we can take them sensitively to some of the more powerful feelings and difficulties.

SOMEONE TO TALK TO

We have looked at our attempts to communicate meaningfully, using words that convey how people are feeling, and how they move up and down the spectrum of those feelings. Whilst this may make us more effective in our communications, there are qualities that people will want to see and experience in us that help them to be comfortable. An exercise to explore this is 'Someone I like talking to.'

In this exercise, participants are asked to spend 5 minutes thinking about a friend or colleague to whom they would talk if they had some difficulty or something good to share. They then make a list of the qualities in that person which make him or her special, for example:

- accessible
- good listener
- non-judgemental
- unlimited time
- comforting
- friendship.

A joint list of these qualities can then be drawn up on the board and used to identify those that apply to the client/counsellor relationship.

This provides some good discussion, for example, on qualities such as open accessibility or friendship. This can bring up the issue of degree of intimacy of the client relationship, and how to separate it from one's personal life. I usually allow 30 minutes to discuss these difficulties in the main group, with any stronger, more difficult problems being explored further in smaller groups for say 10–15 minutes.

BODY LANGUAGE

What your body says about you is not always apparent to you. We all pick up habits that are annoying to others or do not convey what we are trying to say. For example, we may unconsciously tap our foot while someone is being long-winded in his explanation of something. Is the foot tapping an expression of our irritation, or something we do when we have difficulty concentrating? If it is the latter this is our problem and it should not be conveyed in this way.

Longer training sessions (2–3 days) allow some of these communication issues to be explored in more detail. When people have had the opportunity to achieve a rapport with fellow workers this next exercise to explore non-verbal communication can be used. The form shown in Figure 7.3 can be used in two ways. The first is to get people to fill them out themselves, using their own awareness to explore the issues involved in each section, and recording how they see their own strengths and weaknesses. Alternatively over a period of a day or two, especially for people working in pairs, partners can make some observations about each other. The observations made can be both positive and negative, but this is *not* meant to be a demoralizing experience.

Posture
Breathing
Voice
Face
Eyes
Mannerisms
Time response
Anything else significant

Figure 7.3 My body talk.

Some questions that may help in exploring each section are listed below:

- Posture
  - Do you slouch down in the chair?
  - Do you sit huddled and appear motionless to pain and anguish?
  - Does this imply to the client that this is damaging you?
  - Do you sit with arms folded?
- Breathing
  - What do your deep sighs mean to others?
  - Is the way you are breathing a sign of your tension or difficulty with this client or with the material?
- Voice
  - Are there changes in tone or strength?
  - At what pace do words emerge?
  - Is there some pressure of speech?
  - Do regional accents matter?
  - In our attempts to reassure, is our tone patronizing?
- Face
  - Do we have one expression for the whole time?
  - Does our expression convey what we mean?
  - Do we smile? Beware of the fixed smile, particularly if accompanied by the 'there there, it will be all right' words.
  - Mouth and jaw held rigid may indicate tension and anxiety.
- Eyes
  - Do we avoid eye contact?
  - How do we fix our eyes, and remain attentive and relaxed?
  - Are some stares intrusive?
  - Do we know when to look away?
  - Is there a tendency to gaze around the room as though uninterested?
- Mannerisms
  - Your use of hands and body movements may give life and meaning to what you say. Constantly picking something up and putting it down, or dismantling a pen, may irritate, especially if you drop the parts and have to search round for them, or cannot fix it together again.
  - Some mannerisms are your hallmark, or say a lot about you, and are not necessarily negative, e.g. the way you straighten your hair or rest your head on your hands.
- Time response
  - Do you hear things out, or terminate other people's conversation prematurely?
  - Are you able to use your time to give structure to your counselling?
  - Are you able to begin it and take it to an appropriate end?
  - Does an awareness of time elapsing produce other body talk?

- Anything else of significance?
  - Some people may want to discuss other issues here which they feel can cause a distraction from the counselling or a difficulty in rapport. Will that ring through your nose be off-putting to the client? A discussion on prejudice, and how it is dealt with, may follow.

The ability to use the knowledge of body language to communicate effectively and to interpret the other person's non-verbal messages is a very important counselling skill.

SETTING UP STUDY DAYS AND WORKSHOPS

Whilst some free space is necessary for what people bring to these work-shops, some structure does remove anxiety. The exercises or approaches discussed here offer ways of exploring the issues involved in sudden death, and of teaching the skills and theory connected with it. Most people are more comfortable with some direction or structure to work within and larger groups are much more manageable if the day is organized.

A programme sent out earlier will give delegates a chance to consider ideas before the event. These workshops are often not suitable to be taken in part, and people must be prepared to attend fully. If people arrive late and are presented with very sensitive issues, well-defended responses are often the result. Leaving early or missing part of the programme gives people an opportunity to avoid difficulties.

The planned use of the personal material of the participants, or their experiences, in exercises, should be stated explicitly on the programme. The intended use of experiential exercises, as well as a straightforward look at the theory, must be made clear.

All this means that participants will have come voluntarily, and know what may be expected of them, and that their input is vital to the success of the day. They can, of course, opt out of exercises, and the facilitator must be sensitive to people's difficulties and have the resources to deal with them. Most difficulties can be used to reflect the concerns and problems of us all and can allow people the opportunity to care for and support colleagues.

When training people to work with sudden death, the pain and problems of the helper always become apparent. This cannot be avoided. We need to ensure that carers themselves are cared for, not only by those running training sessions but also within the structure of their organizations.

Teaching requires sensitivity to the carers' distress. It will also become apparent that some care workers cannot cope with or tolerate vulner-ability in each other. We are vulnerable, there is no doubt about that, and colleagues can respond to our vulnerability in a way which does not indicate that we are unsuitable, or less of a person. Workshop organizers may be accused of introducing material that is too personal, breaks down carers' defences and causes some stress. The response to this criticism is that clients have a way of doing just that. Working with sudden death is stressful and the next chapter considers how to manage this stress.

Activity 7B

For the group facilitator or teacher: What is the response you fear most from the individual or group? How would you deal with this? What stresses might you experience in this work?

REFERENCES

Lazarus R 1966 Psychological stress and the coping process. McGraw Hill, New York
Wordon J W 1991 Grief counselling and grief therapy. 2nd edn. Tavistock, London
Publications for self-directed learning:
Wright B 1992 Loss and grief. Churchill Livingstone, Edinburgh
Wright B 1992 Communication skills. Churchill Livingstone, Edinburgh

8

Caring for ourselves

Before we consider some of the difficulties of working with sudden death, it is worth clarifying what is meant by stress. Stress is a message that some coping mechanism is required, the signal to mobilize resources. In the previous chapter on training we explored how stress is about excessive internal and external demands and our response to these. What is stressful depends on the way we think about ourselves and the situation we are in. What demands are being made upon us, and what do these demands mean?

THE CONCEPT OF STRESS

The development of the concept of stress has contributed to an under-standing of the nature and causes of disease, as well as to its psychological implications. Basic issues connected with stress have been applied to biological, psychological and social behaviour. R S Lazarus (1966), H Selye (1976), H Wolfe (1950) and W Cannon (1935) are amongst the theorists who have made significant contributions to the development of the concept of stress.

Cannon (1935) examined stress as a causative factor of disease. He described how stresses place pressures on specific mechanisms of the body necessary to maintain a steady state. This state of equilibrium is called homeostasis — maintaining a correct balance of temperature control, fluid and electrolyte balance, nervous system control and immune system response. Cannon viewed disease as a failure to maintain the homeostatic mechanisms under stress.

Wolfe (1950) described stress as a dynamic state within the organism, an internal force produced by external forces. He viewed stress as an interaction between the external environment and the individual.

Past experiences are a contributing factor in determining the response to the stress. Wolfe described a 'protective reaction pattern' — a complex reaction to rid the body of threat, with symbolic and physical threats initiating similar responses. This pattern involves alteration in feeling, body processes and behaviour.

Selye (1976) focused his attention on the biochemical and physiological effects of stress. He described the body's response as non-specific, in that all or most parts of the body must try to adjust to any agent of stress. Selye relates stress to homeostasis, for example he describes shivering as the body's adaptive response to cold stress, the goal being to return the body to its previous steady state.

Selye's General Adaptive Syndrome (GAS) describing stress in all people involves three stages of adaptation:

1. the alarm reaction
2. the stage of resistance
3. the state of exhaustion.

The alarm reaction is the early response of the body's defence mechanism and cannot be maintained for too long or death will follow. The resistance stage leads to homeostasis and survival. The exhaustion stage results from this activity when it is prolonged, and can lead to ageing.

Selye believes that for most short-lived, more manageable stressors, only the first and second stages are apparent. Repeated encounters with the first and second stage lead to people learning to adapt to the environment. Severe exhaustion is only initiated by more serious threat, and it is not experienced as often as the other stages. Selye goes on to say that an individual's adaptability allows him, in all the complexities of life, to resist stress and return to homeostasis. He notes that hereditary factors play some part in stress response/effects.

Lazarus (1966) described how the degree of reaction to a stressor is related to the subjective appraisal each individual makes of the event as being threatening or non-threatening. The Lazarus Cognitive Model of Stress has three phases:

1. appraisal
2. coping
3. outcome.

Appraisal occurs when the stressor and the degree of danger are evaluated. Secondary appraisal involves assessing the availability of adequate coping devices. Direct action, by meeting or avoiding the approaching threat, may be a coping mechanism. The other coping mechanism is to alter the distress felt, by working with the response to the event. The effectiveness of appraisal and coping affects the outcome, that is, the effect the stressor has upon the person.

Stress is an essential component of life, and need not always have negative connotations. The negative aspect of stress could, perhaps, be more accurately described as distress. In working with sudden death we come across both stress and distress.

COPING MECHANISMS

The definitions for coping are many, and as varied as those for adaptation to stress. Some authorities identify coping more readily in the context of crisis, or in adjustment to adverse conditions. It involves problem-solving efforts in situations which are perceived as very important to the individual, and which make demands on his adaptive resources (Lazarus & Folkman 1984); this approach considers coping to be primarily a cognitive process. Levin et al (1978) recognize the relationship between psychosocial and cognitive processes. They define the ultimate goal of coping as the reduction of physiological activity.

In general terms, coping refers to processes or skills used to deal with situations or events which are out of the ordinary for that individual. In the integrated process (using both psychosocial and cognitive processes) 'gut feelings' influence cognition of the need to cope. Stimuli to coping arise in the external environment in the form of physical factors, inter-personal relationships and community, national and international events. Stimuli in the internal environment include thoughts, feelings and physical illness.

For even the most competent amongst us, continued exposure to particularly difficult and emotionally draining situations can result in serious emotional crisis. Crisis work, although valued, can be difficult to tolerate especially as it often covers a wide range of human conditions.

Attending to a bleeding, multiply injured patient, followed by someone with a minor cut of the hand, demands of a nurse some rapid changes in energy and focus. Some clients are demanding, unappreciative, hostile and difficult. Concern about a patient's physical or psychological condition can lead to feelings of frustration at being unable to do more. It is easy in such situations for carers to begin to lose emotional objectivity and control. Carers may be left feeling ineffective and helpless.

Whilst personal responses are a factor identified as a predictor of burn-out in nurses, so also are organizational factors (Hare et al 1988). Concern about the negative effects of stress, and the need to minimize acute distress, has influenced research to identify and analyse the various working environments of nurses (Brunt 1984, Caldwell 1976, Keller 1990, Phipps 1988).

Much of the research literature is anecdotal. There is a lot of discussion concerning deaths, violence, pain and hostility. However, a survey by Burns et al 1983 identified organizational issues as a greater stressor than the events themselves, with Unit management being cited as the greatest source of stress. Care issues ranked second to inadequate staffing and inexperienced medical staff in this study.

The results of another study (Hawley 1992) show that although stress relates to a variety of sources, inadequate staffing and resources, and non-nursing tasks have a serious impact on nurses' ability to provide quality care. Another major source of distress though is confronting families in crisis.

In dealing with the crisis of sudden death, nurses in particular run a higher risk of personal stress than either the general public or other human service workers (Mahoney 1991). Some recommendations from Mahoney's study are that in the curriculum for emergency nurses, staff educators should include recognizing burnout, coping skills and awareness of post-trauma symptoms after these incidents.

Emergency nurses, in anecdotal discussion, talk enthusiastically about their work and how they value its diversity. Although little has been written about personality types in nursing, this attitude appears to conflict with the needs of the personality types we know.

According to Atkins & Piazza (1987), the majority of emergency nurses are independent, diligent, task-orientated and enjoy working alone; this personality type does not appear to fit in with Accident & Emergency nursing. These same individuals were able to make rapid decisions, plan, order, control and remain with the task; there is, however, a tendency to be stubborn, inflexible, unadaptable and judgemental. Accident & Emergency nurses exhibiting these characteristics strongly will have difficulty working with the bereaved. For example, the nature of bereaved people's responses mean the carer has to be flexible, non-judgemental, and adaptable to chaos and disorder. An inability to stay with this leads to frustration and helplessness, and, ultimately, to burnout.

The knowledge that certain personality characteristics can affect work performance may help in selection of staff, or in training to develop appropriate approaches to crisis work.

Although we may value the importance of caring for others, there may be a cost to us personally. How we manage these demands depends on our tolerance of what we are confronted with, and whether or not we have any control or mastery over the situation. If we can reduce or minimize the disorder in the situation, some order or control will result. Control is a word used often in training sessions, for coping is not necessarily about success but about change and our efforts to manage or control it. The outcome may not be what we want, but we may be satisfied with our input in order to alter it, or we may adapt to it. So stress may be the mechanism through which we find ways of coping with something difficult.

GETTING HELP

The simple response of listening requires skills discussed earlier in the book, and done well can be very effective. Finding a colleague with whom you can talk and share difficulties is a well-used and caring response. This involves self-disclosure, and requires trust and the ability to glimpse the 'person' behind the professional role (Wright 1992).

How the story is told and heard, and how the story-teller hears his own story, is emphasized in other work on coping with stressful incidents (McKechnie 1993). Talking helps to clarify and identify difficulties, and often alters the speaker's perception of the event. Although listening is a basic and perhaps simple skill, its value should not be underestimated.

It has long been recognized that certain critical incidents may be difficult for student nurses to tolerate. After such incidents, we have sought them out to check whether they were managing their feelings. This follow-up is important for both new and experienced staff.

IDENTIFICATION

For most people, an encounter with a death that intimately concerns them occurs only a few times in their lives. Some people will talk of hearing of several deaths recently, but these may have no profound implications for them; they merely know of them.

Working with sudden death means one encounter after another, and an intimate knowledge of its effect on loved ones. The carer will often ask herself what effect this abnormal exposure to death is having upon her. Other people will ask her how she copes with it all, perhaps hoping to hear of some secret formula that protects her from it.

Activity 8A

Consider how the stress models discussed will help you to have a greater understanding of the stress experienced by people working with sudden death.

We sometimes talk of putting ourselves in another person's place to try to imagine what her needs are and to increase our sensitivity — this is called identification. If we do not have the ability to disengage from identification and to remember that:

'I am not you and the feelings are yours not mine'

we are in trouble. We can become burdened with emotion that does not belong to us and will be less effective as a carer.

Identification may occur because of similar life styles, sex, age, occupation or appearance of the client. The identification then becomes a mechanism by which the carer patterns his personality on that of the client, assuming that person's qualities, characteristics and responses. We need to be constantly sensitive to this possibility occurring; it is to be avoided.

DISPLACEMENT

This tendency can also add to the burden of the carer unless he has some insights into it. We came across displacement in Chapter 2 when exploring the issue of advocacy for the bereaved person in health care settings. A relative of the bereaved may ask:

'How can you ask her [the bereaved person] to see the body; you are adding to her distress.'

They might really mean:

'Asking her to do that will distress her and add to my distress, and I will be left to pick up the pieces.'

Displacement is the shift of an emotion from the person it was directed towards, to another person (or object), usually neutral or less dangerous. This is not only a difficulty on impact of sudden death, but often arises in bereavement counselling.

Carers need to be aware of the difference between displacement and projection. Projection is when the client attributes his own thoughts or impulses to another person. When this other person is the carer, the carer can find it very stressful. This is particularly so if there is marked anger or aggression.

'At the hospital, at the time of a sudden death, I was discussing with the deceased's companion the handing over of valuables and jewellery. She became very angry and accused me of suggesting that she was immediately going to gain from his death. This was her response when I told her I could not hand over a large sum of money found on the patient since she had informed me she was not a relative.

She said the money was hers, and despite my saying I was not refuting that but needed evidence, and that I had to go through the correct procedures, more projections occurred. She went on to say that I thought she only cared for this man to extract money from him, that I thought she was cold-blooded and criminal.

In a powerful outpouring of emotion, it became apparent that these were also the thoughts of some of his relatives. I had no reason at all to suspect her motives, and was only trying to explain the intricacies of the procedure for handing over money.'

A woman, whose husband died after throwing himself from a tall building, said shortly after she was told of his death:

"You think I drove him to it, don't you? I have no one else if that's what you think. I don't suppose you have ever got it wrong, said the wrong thing and regretted it. All right, you think I'm a bitch."

All this anger and bitterness can make the carer, against whom it is directed, feel very defensive and vulnerable. This causes even more problems. The defensiveness can be interpreted as confirmation that you do indeed feel how they thought you did, when nothing could be further from the truth. If you respond with 'Why do you think that?', the projection may then be generalized and made less personal: 'That's what people will think, I know.' Generalizations are more easily worked with and less confrontational.

It is very useful to the care worker to have some knowledge of coping mechanisms, identification and displacement as these are common responses to acute distress. There will be some days, however, when a worker feels very vulnerable, and may forget these insights. Displacement, in particular, can be painful, accusatory, judgemental, and make the carer suddenly feel ineffectual, or perhaps angry. A sensitive colleague may remind us, when we feel like this, of what is going on.

THE PERSONAL TOLL OF CARING

Caring may take its toll both emotionally and physically, and caregivers themselves can become the casualties. Bailey (1985), in his evaluation of the research in this field as well as his own work, considers that nurses and doctors are more at risk than those they care for. This group, and other allied health professionals, are perhaps more exactingly exposed to great suffering.

Ethical issues about resuscitation measures being discontinued are usually not a problem but, occasionally, team members will disagree on the timing of cessation of attempts. The final decision usually lies with the doctors, but nurses have to put that decision into practice with or without them (Melia & Boyd 1994). Nurses working in critical care will experience being surrounded by people and activity, only to be left alone with a bloody and broken body when all this activity has ceased. Issues of power and control may be of great concern to these nurses.

Julie had worked in Emergency for 3 years. Despite its demands and difficulties, she got something from its variety and unpredictability.

It was a usual Saturday night with its quota of road traffic accidents and victims of assault and crime. The patients and friends were noisy, and at times disruptive. Julie had grown to be quite comfortable with this.

She was summoned to the resuscitation room where a 17-year-old youth had arrived with two stab wounds to the abdomen. He was shocked, gasping for breath, and had classical signs of air hunger. There were a lot of people in the room, all making demands. Intravenous lines were quickly established, blood sent to the lab for group- and cross-matching, cardiac monitoring begun and a central venous line established. Continuous blood pressure and pulse monitoring indicated a fast-deteriorating condition. He was bleeding to death despite vigorous efforts to save him.

Staff were becoming impatient with each other, some were beginning to shout if instruments or equipment did not just suddenly appear. Fear and frustration at losing the fight to save him were being expressed in this way.

The decision was made to do an emergency laparotomy. His abdomen was opened and the enormity of his wounds became apparent — severe damage to the arteries and liver. Finding this, in the blood-filled cavity of the abdomen, took some time — time he did not have. The patient was by now ventilated and having external cardiac massage. Shouts for more of this and that were heard, but it was too late.

The boy died and a decision to abandon the resuscitation was made. The patient's abdomen was sewn up, he was disconnected from the monitors, and the intubation tubes removed. The hissing of the oxygen ceased, as did the suctions. The high activity came to a halt, and several staff left the room.

Julie looked at her colleague, then at the still, lifeless body waiting to be washed. The room was quiet. 'This is the end of the line,' Julie thought. 'This is what you are left with when you don't succeed, and when people fight and kill each other.' Julie said to her friend: 'Do we know who he is? We don't even have a name. I wonder if his Mum and Dad are waiting for him to come home.' As they washed his damaged young body, they both unashamedly cried.

At times, care workers are left powerless and helpless. They may carry physical and emotional burdens that are too much to bear, and the cost of caring results in burnout.

BURNOUT

Burnout, in the caring or helping professions, affects both client and carer. The client sees or experiences a care worker who is no longer committed, lacks the energy for the work, or fails to see any useful outcome. From the client's point of view, there is a lack of concern for them, or for the job. From the carer's point of view it may be that the complete reverse of this has produced the burnout. Over-commitment, over-concern, over-investment of energy and resources has left little for self. The loss of idealism, purpose and energy, which is so necessary and seen as so vital in caring for the bereaved, is a cause for grief.

Carers can become overwhelmed with sadness for the predicament they are in, and may well display all those emotional responses we identified earlier in the client. Anger, denial, crying and withdrawal may well be overt symptoms in the burntout professional.

Because carers tend to want to deny that they are as vulnerable as clients, intervention may be late or difficult. It may seem that we cannot stay with our own vulnerability because to do so makes us so aware of our own fragility that we would be unable to function effectively. Nevertheless, we must not be so well-defended that we fail to care for ourselves. It is not inevitable that working with sudden death will produce burnout. If carers need to be defended enough to work effectively with it, and I am not sure they do, they must have some mechanism whereby colleagues are able to respond to them, and intervene at the appropriate time, before they feel damaged.

Burnout is expressed in various physical and emotional forms as outlined next:

- Physical signs
  - fatigue, loss of energy and drive, feelings of weariness and exhaustion
  - coughs, colds, headaches that take a long time to clear up
  - nausea, indigestion, colicky pain, diarrhoea, constipation
  - disturbed sleep, waking tired
  - working all night in our dreams
  - difficulty getting off to sleep or waking early
  - suddenly waking remembering some incident at work, or something we have forgotten to do
  - itching, rashes, dry or oily skin
  - shortness of breath or hyperventilating with tachycardia
  - wheezing
  - general malaise, aches and pains, unexplained loss of energy.

There is usually perplexity and preoccupation with the above symptoms, and an underlying anxiety that they indicate some serious, debilitating illness. A lot of time can be spent pondering over the nature of the illness and discussing its outcome.

- Emotional signs
  - emotionally labile, i.e. oversensitive, irritable, easily moved to tears and marked distress
  - quickly in touch with anger, or moved from irritability to anger; a need to blame others, or point the finger
  - surprise at the sudden emergence of this anger with apparently little justified stimulus; an inappropriateness about it
  - strong feelings of sadness or hopelessness; this might take on a global aspect, such as being fearful for mankind and its inhumanity or self-destructiveness
  - outbursts of screaming and shouting; lashing out
  - suspicion that easily becomes overt paranoia; thoughts that people are talking about you, particularly to do with your effectiveness or lack of control; leading to thoughts of going mad
  - avoiding clients/patients and commitments to caring for them
  - finding trivial reasons for not encountering them
  - becoming bogged down in paperwork or bureaucracy; difficulty concentrating, or not wanting to; lack of energy, lethargy; difficulty staying with the focus.

'Work is one long struggle. At our place it's a constant struggle to keep in with the boss and keep enough credibility for her deputy's job, which will soon become vacant. She's the lucky one, leaving soon.

I get fed up with teaching new staff and dealing with the endless number of people doing research into this and that, and asking questions. Soon it will be school-kids for work experience. As if we didn't have enough to do. Someone is always coming up with something new, some idea to streamline or improve the organization. It is all a constant change and a hassle.

I want to be left alone just to get on with my own work. I'm not sure if I like it any more.'

It is not enough just to know what burnout is. We should also know what can be done about it. Having decided that working with sudden death is beginning to overwhelm you, there are some suggestions that may afford some help. Preventing further pain or distress to yourself may demand some change that is frightening. When the dissatisfaction is removed, we need to be sure we want what is left, or that we can move in a direction that offers something new and satisfying.

One of the problems for nurses working in critical care is failure to cope with the deaths, particularly of young people. Critical care areas also have a lot of technology, excessive demands for beds, and often poor resources and staff shortages. Manley (1986), an intensive care nurse teacher, identified workload and environment as major stressors for intensive care nurses. Next were emotional issues relating to death and severe illness. Following on from these two were interstaff stress and responsibility for life and death decisions.

Pot-Mees (1987), in discussing the stress in bone marrow transplant units, describes how the person-centred 'holistic' approach to nursing care, whilst having its rewards, means a closer encounter with the relatives' fears, frustrations and anger as well as the rewards of seeing patients recover. This new and challenging role means the nurse is more vulnerable and is subject to more stress than in the past. Working with high technology and the more concrete issues, and then having to make a shift to dealing with someone's feelings, is not an easy transition to make. Pot-Mees suggests the difficulty and personal risk of working in this way may be alleviated by good support systems, outside distractions and personal insight.

Working with the immediate issues of sudden death in hospitals over a long period of time requires carers to maintain a personal belief in themselves and their effectiveness in this situation, to believe in the strength, resources and resilience of people, and to have good support systems. Someone having difficulty with these, may consider the following:

- further training
- outside interests
- a change of work
- support systems
- adjusting expectations.

Re-education or further education

In working with sudden death, we need some affirmation of the outcome of the work in both the immediate and the long term. If we only work with its immediate effects we need to be aware of the long-term progress. Most people find resources to handle a sudden bereavement, and we may need to be reminded of this. Those who work with the long-term effects need to see that people do make progress after its awful impact. This awareness helps us to see that we are only one cog in the caring wheel; the burden is not entirely ours. Regular time out to hear about research and ways of working with sudden death are essential.

Life outside work

Sport, leisure, courses, and other ways of being distracted, are essential. Many critical care, high-tech units arrange theatre/concert visits, barbecues and other social events. Relaxation through yoga, massage and aromatherapy can work extremely well for some.

Ask for a move

A move from well-worn routines and to something less demanding may be necessary. This may involve a change of hours, and may be all we need to see things differently. Working with a different type of client or with a longer or shorter transaction are options to consider. The alternative to a move is working for a change in the existing situation.

Encouraging support systems

It may help to set up support groups within the area of work and allow time for this in the working day. It is important to care for and support one another — we tend not to recognize our own needs.

Difficulties and expected outcomes

Some patients, clients and relatives will not match up to our expectations of them. We are dealing with people, and must acknowledge their right to reject what we have to offer. Some people have resources within themselves or elsewhere to support them with their difficulties.

Sometimes, planned ways of working will have to be changed or disrupted. If we fail to recognize this, or become inflexible to the needs of people, we will feel let down and become disillusioned.

POST-TRAUMATIC STRESS DISORDER

The study by Durham et al (1985) on the emotional response to the impact of disaster of medical personnel, police, firemen, paramedics and rescue workers found that 80% had at least one symptom of post-traumatic stress disorder (PTSD). On-the-scene staff had significantly more symptoms than did hospital staff. This study was based on questionnaires returned after an apartment building explosion in Greenville, North Carolina. Kolb (1986) cites the long-term excessive mortality of those who served in the military during the Vietnam conflict; suicide and road traffic accidents were increased in this section of the population. Kolb recommends that serious consideration be given to reports of the impaired psychosocial and health status of these men.

Certain responses can be identified as associated with disaster syndrome or post-traumatic stress disorder, although any individual's response to a traumatic event is valid. Whilst many of our clients have suffered a traumatic life experience, so have emergency rescue personnel and people working in critical care. Once an unmanageable level for stress is reached in these workers, recognized patterns of response emerge as outlined next.

Initial phase — impact and denial

Despite the media commonly showing an overt, noisy and dramatic response to trauma, the reality is usually the opposite. The response is often flat and full of denial, apparently lacking in awareness of the true nature of the event. The immediate focus is on survival. It could be argued that the denial is of benefit to the worker in that it prevents excessive fears overwhelming him.

Intermediate phase — confrontation and disorder

In this phase the worker recognizes what has happened, and is clearly confronting the disaster. Sleep disturbances, nightmares and dreams become a worrying part of this phase. Preoccupation with the event, flashbacks and intrusive thoughts are usually a feature. People become hypersensitive to sudden loud noises or bangs; you may notice this on an orthopaedic ward, where there are victims of road traffic accidents.

Being dependent on others makes the worker angry, and the anger is often directed towards colleagues or authority and the organization. This anger can have a rebellious, adolescent nature about it. At the opposite end of this scale of responses is passive non-compliance.

Depression and guilt are often components of this anger. Elation at survival soon becomes the opposite — guilt at survival. A worker who becomes particularly helpful or cooperative, never complaining or showing dissent, may be making amends for having survived.

Colleagues can help the worker by assisting him to begin the process of grieving and coping. The worker may need his colleagues' permission to express such feelings, especially the men, who may feel foolish about showing sad emotions.

Final phase — readjustment and recovery

Here, the worker looks towards the future, and leaves the state of 'sick' person behind. He begins to take an interest in others, and in the community at large. He gradually loses his dependency and takes control of his own life. Realizing what he is now capable of doing, he becomes hopeful of making the adjustment.

In summary, the psychological sequelae to a traumatic event are:

- Initial phase — impact and denial
- Intermediate phase — confrontation and disorder
- Final phase — readjustment and recovery.

Colleagues can help the affected carer by having insight into these phases and recognizing where she is. They can help her through the phases, to reach her full potential again.

We have looked at ways of working with and addressing symptoms of burnout and post-traumatic stress disorder in the individual. We now move on to setting up support systems within an organization.

STRESS DEBRIEFING

The recent spate of disasters has highlighted how the carer can become the victim. We have begun to recognize the phenomenon of bystander bereavement, i.e. not being a direct victim but witnessing a painful or traumatic event. Working with sudden death may be just that; witnessing or being overwhelmed by the anguish of the people, at the time or later, and not having the resources or ability to prevent this somehow consuming us. The carer then becomes the victim.

In their study of one disaster, Durham et al (1985) found that 70% of the workers reported intrusive, repetitive thoughts about the event, and 15% reported intrusive dreams and depression. Workers who had been at the scene were more likely to experience these difficulties. Successful adjustment in this study involved focusing on the meaning of the event, gaining mastery over the situation, and preparing mentally for a recurrence of the event. Each of these tasks is an issue for workers in any sudden death.

People working with sudden death frequently report how surprised they are at their own calmness at the time. Woodruff (1989) found that only hours and days later does the stress become apparent. Vivid dreams, shaking, anxiety or not wanting to return home were some common responses. This study concluded that staff counsellors should be available not only for disasters but also for everyday hospital events that cause stress.

In investigations over the past 2 years I have talked to people in the UK, Australia and the USA about structured ways of debriefing critical incidents (Wright 1989). Some of these incidents involved the death and injury of large numbers of people. Others, whilst not involving large numbers, concerned the sudden, maybe traumatic deaths of one or more people. These incidents all demand from the health service and other personnel a sudden outpouring of resources both physically and emotionally. They are described as 'critical incidents'.

CRITICAL INCIDENTS

A critical incident is any situation, faced by emergency personnel, that causes them to experience unusually strong emotional reactions. These feelings have the potential to interfere with their ability to function at the time or later. Critical incidents result in some characteristic physical and psychological symptoms. These are quite normal and common responses to an abnormal event.

Some carers react immediately after the event or within a few hours or days. In some cases, though, it is weeks or months before a reaction appears. The signs and symptoms of the stress reaction may last for a few days and some support and understanding will often help the feelings dissipate. For others, the event is so painful that more structured assistance is required. This is carried out most effectively by a peer group member with some skills in debriefing.

Critical incident stress debriefing (CISD) requires a facilitator with good working knowledge of stress and counselling. Mitchell (1983) states that its value should not be underestimated as it prolongs the careers of personnel. This prevents resources having to be used on training new personnel and retains expertise.

Hearing too many expressions of pain, and witnessing too many broken bodies, may take its toll. The three procedures used to alleviate the stress of critical incidents are: defusing, demobilization and debriefing. These are discussed in detail next.

Defusing

Defusing may best be described as a short type of crisis intervention for critical care staff and other emergency personnel. It is particularly suited to people who are required to act and control situations. The aim of the defusing is to make the incident less harmful to those involved. This is achieved by helping to restore control and by providing immediate support and assistance. It should reduce tension, focus on strengths and help carers to regain emotional control. This focus on skills helps to ensure a return to normal functioning and the start of the process of recovery. A return to cognitive functioning enables the person to think rather than react.

The facilitator or interventionist maintains a low profile in defusing procedures. The people involved are encouraged to take the lead and do the talking. Once this process begins, most people become more spontaneous. Defusing is short-term, and the parameters are set by the people themselves. They take charge of the level of emotional ventilation. They take it to where they want and then return to normal functioning.

Nurses will recognize the report or handover time as an example of a defusing period. Although the whole shift is to be reported on, or a group of patients in a certain order, any critical incident should receive the immediate attention. Until all the details of this event have been shared, it is difficult to discuss other events effectively. If attempts are made to curtail the disclosure this will cause it to emerge later. For any group of workers involved with a critical incident, time and attention are necessary to allow it to be laid to rest.

A satisfactory conclusion occurs when all the facts and feelings about the event have been shared. By putting it to rest in this way, a return to normal functioning is achieved. Key information is given to everyone so that the whole episode leaves no questions or perplexity.

The first 24 hours after an event will see the denial response at its most powerful. This form of insulation may be necessary, and should not be viewed as unhealthy. However, it may be appropriate to view denial in the long-term as unhealthy. A gentle approach to denial is always necessary. In the impact phase denial may provide some safety, or a retreat from the pain and distress. This can be the safety valve needed for the moment. If it is persisting, this can be worked with later.

Facilitators must make a mental note of who may need more than defusing, and offer further help. A simple but powerful input at this time is to thank workers for their contribution and to remind them that distress at such events is normal — it is the event and not they who are abnormal. Questions such as 'What happened there?' will elicit facts about the incident, and 'What did you think about it?' encourages the sharing of thoughts. The facilitator should reassure people that their answers are very normal. After these fairly safe disclosures, those involved can begin to move more cautiously into what made the event different, and what was the worst part about it. They will need most help to manage their feelings. Finally, a question or statement that brings the span of duty to an end should close the defusing:

'Who will be at home when you get there?'

or

'It is now time to draw this to an end and for you to go home'.

Remember, defusing is a short act of discharge designed to help people return to cognitive functioning. It may need to be followed up.

Demobilization

Demobilization provides personnel with a structured end to a span of duty. Large-scale incidents benefit the most from this approach, so a room is needed for large numbers of personnel. People entering the room should, ideally, be able to obtain a drink. As they will be tired, they will expect to be detained for 15 minutes at the most. The person leading the demobilization should have as much accurate, factual information as is possible. There is no place for rumours or guesses.

Everyone involved should be ordered to attend the demobilization, it is not just for the vulnerable or sensitive, or those who think they need it. It is for the whole team, and it should be made clear that they all need it. Demobilization is designed to facilitate an end to a stressful working period. The aims of demobilization are as follows:

- to regain emotional control and cognitive functioning, and reduce tension
- to focus on strengths and skills
- to re-evaluate the incident and receive some factual information
- to begin the recovery process and leave behind some of the stress
- to begin to be educated by the critical incident.

The process of demobilization may be begun by the leader saying something like: 'At 15.30 today a multiple accident occurred on the southbound carriageway of the ....' All available information is then given as to rescue services and emergency personnel involved, numbers, types of casualties, and hospitals involved. Because different critical care staff may have looked after different members of a family, information about the condition of them all will be useful.

This exercise helps to complete the picture for staff involved, and to prevent them taking away unanswered questions. The goals may seem similar to those of defusing; the difference is that demobilization has a more definite time limit, the leader is clearly designated, and participation by staff is limited. Staff are told that further help will be given later, and where this may be obtained.

The focus in demobilization is primarily on cognitive functioning rather than emotional ventilation. The workers should be able to leave with a good knowledge of all available facts, and an overall perception of the event. Again, the expression of thanks and their dismissal helps the personnel to bring the span of duty and the event to a conclusion.

At this stage they need to focus on their own resources. If the demobilization is a positive experience, they will return for defusing or debriefing. The leader will still have to be available after the dismissal for people with immediate difficulties they cannot resolve themselves.

Large-scale events involve many people, and it is necessary to provide useful information in a short time to the maximum number of people. They will need reassurance that they did a good job, but that the event was abnormal and for this reason further help may be needed.

Critical Incident Stress Debriefing (CISD)

This is a more formal type of debriefing, and should be done by someone with knowledge of counselling skills, stress management and, if possible, with a knowledge of the working procedure in an emergency situation. For example, if an emergency nurse is being debriefed, then an emergency nurse with the aforementioned skills would be ideal.

Formal CISDs take place 24–48 hours after the event. Mitchell (1983) says that a group meeting is most useful first, followed by individual debriefings. The individual debriefing has six phases, which take a total of 3–5 hours.

Phase 1

After introductions, the rules about confidentiality are explained. The client needs an absolute assurance that no details of the debriefing will be divulged. If he feels guilty, particularly of some sin of omission rather than commission, he needs to be sure it will not be used against him.

Phase 2

The counsellor asks the client to give some details of personal involvement in the incident. He could describe what he saw, what he did, and what he heard and smelled. Anticipation of what will be encountered on arrival at the scene can be very distressing. He will be asked about how he received the message to attend, and about his thoughts prior to arriving on the scene.

Phase 3

When all this factual information has been dealt with the counsellor can go on to ask how he felt. This could centre around the questions:

'How did you feel at the time?'
'How are you feeling now?'
'Have you ever felt like this before?'

These questions usually produce a great outpouring of feelings; frustration, fear, guilt, anger and ambivalence are common. Many apologize that the feelings are about what appears to be a trivial aspect of the event. They need reassurance that because it is important to them it needs to be expressed.

Phase 4

This phase concerns changes that have occurred both at the event and afterwards. The client will be asked about the impact it has had on his life, and what effect it will have on his future. The discussion should focus not only on the work situation, but on how it has affected him at home.

Phase 5

This phase is used to teach something about stress and how individuals respond. Information about common physical symptoms, sleep patterns and emotional reactions can be described. Again, the emphasis is on what happens to normal people, and that it was the event he was involved in that was abnormal and distressing.

Phase 6

This phase brings the debriefing to an end. It is aptly called the re-entry phase, because if debriefing has been effective, the client will be able to work again effectively. Hopefully, he will have discharged any distress, learned something about himself, and have been finally reassured.

When all outstanding issues are dealt with, the debriefing is clearly at an end. Any loose ends will have been tied up, and some people will talk of a plan of action which is now possible since they have been able to disengage from the critical incident.

Follow-up

After 6 months, the personnel may meet again as a group, but this is not always necessary. Some problem may have emerged, or re-emerged, because of the event. Individuals with long-term problems may also be identified here. Some will have been put in touch with some past conflict that compounded the difficulty. They may need further professional expertise or advice.

Many carers, social workers, crisis teams, as well as doctors and nurses, face people and incidents related to a disastrous event. Other incidents, whilst not a major disaster, are unusual or an exacerbation of a daily event. A nurse, for example, may deal with a death from a road traffic accident daily, or quite frequently. Where there are two or three deaths in the same family or accident, the nurse will have to mobilize all her physical and emotional resources to deal with this. This can truly be described as a critical incident — it has the potential to leave the nurse feeling damaged and ineffective.

If people working with sudden death can be freed from guilt, anxiety and some frustration as well as other physical symptoms, that is good. It is good for their work, their efficiency and their effectiveness. Having to replace good personnel is a waste of resources and time.

With shortages of time, resources and personnel, we may have a long wait for debriefing to take place. Stress debriefing needs to be built into the structure and space of departments working with sudden deaths. It must be part of work schedules, and not an afterthought or something to be squeezed into too few hours in a day.

Some of the principles of debriefing are very simple, and this may lead to underestimation of its value. If it is used well, there is every likelihood that some overwhelming and potentially destructive feelings will assume manageable proportions.

THE SUPPORT GROUP

Another support for people working with sudden death is to set time aside each week for the sole purpose of airing difficulties in a group. If this is done in work time, it is an acknowledgement by management that the work is stressful, that there is a real need to share, confront, comfort and support each other. This results in an effective and more cohesive team.

A multidisciplinary team recognizes that everyone's contribution is valued and that common fears, anxieties and problems are shared. The group work endorses to other people and departments the value of the team's interaction, and is a good role model. It will need to be made clear that there are benefits in sharing in this way. Many will wonder how safe it is to expose themselves to a group. It must be emphasized that the aim is to support each other, increase empathy and resolve emotional issues that occur due to the emotional nature of the work. The sole aim of the support group is to care for the staff. It is not to make them accountable, or increase their effectiveness, though the latter may be one of the spin-offs.

The support group is a place to go and be yourself, with all your vulnerability. Hopefully, people will find solutions to problems and will be able to air feelings and views in safety. It may be necessary to define the aims of the group clearly and in a written form. Discussion could begin with people's expectations of the group. Another session may be spent discussing the ground rules of the group; anxiety will be reduced if everyone has a copy.

Some ground rules for group sessions (Gendlin & Beebe 1968) are as follows:

- Everyone who is here belongs here just because he is here and for no other reason.
- For each person, what is true is determined by what is in him, what he directly feels and finds making sense in himself and the way he lives inside himself.
- Our first purpose is to make contact with each other. Everything else we want or need comes second.
- We try to be as honest as possible and to express ourselves as we really are and really feel — just as much as we can.
- We listen for the person inside, living and feeling.
- We listen to everyone.
- The group leader is responsible for two things only: he protects the belonging of every member, and he protects their being heard if this is getting lost.
- Realism — if we know things are a certain way, we do not pretend they are not that way.

- What we say here is confidential. No one will repeat anything said here outside the group, unless it concerns only himself. This applies not just to obviously private things but to everything. If the individual concerned wants others to know something, he can always tell them himself.
- Decisions made by the group need everyone to take part in some way.
- New members become members because they walk in and remain. Whoever is here belongs.

The overall philosophy of these rules emphasizes how increased empathy can be achieved. They offer some clear guidelines about what is and what is not allowed.

Any organizational difficulties of the group, and a look at its aims and values, should be undertaken after 4–6 weeks.

The group facilitator will need specific skills, as well as a thorough knowledge of support group processes and dynamics. Part of the group facilitator's role will be to offer information, though offering too much information, and with no thought for the timing, will cause people to drop out. Facilitating the group will be mostly concerned with sharing ideas, rather than with dispensing information.

Burnard (1987) suggests that verbal intervention, focusing on three different aspects of time, will be useful to the facilitator:

- clarifying recent talk
- developing current talk
- initiating further talk.

This framework is an easily retained way of managing the people in a support group.

Group work should not be regarded as an economy of effort. It is an effective way of offering support and strength. It is not a way into individual counselling, or a substitute for this. Joining a group is an opportunity to give support as well as to receive it. This may cause carers some problems; we find difficulty in receiving help, and even compliments. On the other hand, we may take offered help although we do not need it, for fear of hurting the other person's feelings. We can be so defensive about being offered help that we reject it for reasons that are unfounded. We may, for example, find encouragement patronizing, especially if people use inappropriate words or phrases like:

'You have done that well.'
'What a good girl.'

Forming support groups that only deal with a crisis denies the long-term difficulties of caring for people who are suddenly bereaved, and the toll it can take on staff. Space must therefore be made for these groups to meet in work time on a regular basis. The frequency will depend on the amount of work that involves sudden deaths.

Anxiety that sometimes people will have little to bring or say, or that they will be frantically searching for problems to make the support group work, is usually unfounded. If the group facilitator makes it clear that good, positive, useful experiences can be brought to the group, this removes the idea that it is just for an outpouring of difficulties. The group may simply want to sit and say quietly, away from the pressure of the work, how much they value each other, and their work, and why.

Staff counsellors

Some hospitals and organizations have made counsellors accessible to staff. More organizations have made outside counsellors available. Staff may contact the counsellor, who is independent of the organization, and may visit the counsellor away from the place of work. For some people, this is the only safe way of receiving help, and this approach recognizes that fact. My anxiety about outside counselling is that it puts the problems far away from the organization. By not having a resident staff counsellor in the vicinity of the work area itself, a major problem could be hidden away.

Supervision of carers and counsellors

Counsellors in any setting have long valued the concept and practice of supervision. Any carer who is very defensive about this must have her practice brought into question. Supervision involves working with someone who is known for having skills, knowledge and experience in the practice of counselling. The supervisor is often senior in terms of years of experience in counselling. Supervision is distinguished from consultation by its ongoing process and the degree of intimacy with the supervisor.

One of the roles of the supervisor is to ensure that the counsellor or carer has the ability to work with the difficulties of the client. The nature of the relationship should provide an opportunity for personal and professional growth, but it is not in itself a therapeutic relationship.

Assisting the counsellor/carer to process usefully what she sees and hears, and how she responds to it, is very confronting and may produce tension and some stress. This can and should be reduced to a working and productive level. It may involve the supervisor discussing the carer/counsellor's expectations about herself.

There are parallel experiential tasks in the supervisory and the therapeutic relationships. A working process, and the questions of what is productive, and how to establish rapport, are usefully explored in this way. The supervisor should be aware that there will be opportunities for role modelling. The carer/counsellor's receptiveness to feedback and its outcome is important. The supervision may help to clarify immediate client problems and decision-making, which then has a direct impact on the client. In an overview of a period of supervision, you may see its indirect impact on the client.

Although the accountability aspect of supervision seems a threat to some, it should be seen as a safeguard for both the client's and carer/ counsellor's interests. It is often apparent in these supervisory periods if the carer's stress is becoming intolerable. Supervision is a way of caring for the carer.

CONCLUSION

There is no way of working through the intervention skills needed in sudden death, without experiencing the stress of it all. Chapter 1 looked at some structured ways of working with sudden death designed to help restore order to a chaotic, disordered episode. This approach helps me to organize my thoughts more usefully when there is pain and disorder all around. Later chapters reviewed the immediate needs of the bereaved family. In immediate care, a nurturing role, providing safety, makes the carer feel useful, and may dissipate whatever stress they feel. Considering the long-term implications of care gives carers some insight into the value of what they do; this is much needed when we are struggling with the job.

To prepare ourselves for the stress, we looked at responses that can incapacitate carers. This will remove some of the perplexity or difficulty of being confronted with these responses on the job. Armed with some knowledge we feel less defenceless. Carers need to be educated and trained for the work. However, in the search for knowledge about working with sudden death, we should realize that whatever way people respond, it is a valid response for them; there is no right or wrong about it, and we must not judge them.

In theory, then, after all this information we should have arrived at a position of greater strength. There is, however, a problem with this and we have already discussed it. These thoughts, theories and structures to work with are for the benefit of the clients. Carers often have different values for themselves:

Ann was recognized within her Emergency department as having a caring manner when dealing with relatives. Whilst she had to have all the skills of a critical care nurse, her particular forté was caring for distressed relatives and the emotional distress in the patient.

Over the years she had gained so much from these people, both in knowledge and in an increase in her own skills. If she knew some members of staff had difficulty with this, she would offer to take work from them, or talk to them afterwards about how they coped and what they had learned. She often reflected on how she walked into outrageously painful situations and attempted to begin something useful, and what it was doing to her. She felt she had something to give and to gain.

For the past 6 months, however, she felt that this had altered. She seemed to be giving more than she gained. There were times when she resented being asked for help by other members of staff; but this was natural, she thought. Recently it had been worse than this — worse because her response was more extreme and worse because she did not realize what was happening. At least previously she had thought her resentment a natural response. Now she had no idea that her response was anger, accusation and bitterness.

Some days it was painfully apparent. When a friend and colleague could not cope with the parents of a teenager dying from a motor cycle accident, she had the following advice and suggestions to offer her:

'Perhaps you are in the wrong job. If you can't stand the heat, why are you here? You are no use to them like this. You have to be strong. If you are after promotion it will not look very good for you.'

These words were coming from Ann — Ann who was usually so outraged when others responded in this way. Resentfully, she went to care for these clients and in her anger and sure knowledge of what they wanted, failed to hear what they were saying to her. She had a recipe of skills that would suit their every need, and she forgot how defenceless and at the mercy of others, people in this position were.

A few days later she was complaining how tired she felt, and how the job was playing havoc with her back, and the rushed meals were giving her indigestion. Her monologue was interrupted by a man shouting in the next room. She knew he was the man whose daughter had taken an overdose, and who was complaining at the length of time she had been kept waiting for treatment.

Ann immediately bemoaned the fact that staff nowadays were so young and inexperienced and not firm enough with people: these people need to be kept in their place, who do they think they are? After all, the girl brought this on herself. The father was probably feeling guilty about not caring for his daughter properly. Ann had not met the man or his daughter, but she immediately assumed she knew what it was about.

Two weeks later during the coffee break, a tired-looking Ann told the whole staff room how much the job had changed. People were too well cared for these days. They expected you to do everything for them. We cannot go on giving more and more without more help. Ann went on to say how people at the top had no idea about what was going on.

A few days later she was again late coming off duty. She decided it was better to sort out the complicated things yourself, in case it all went wrong.

You are only left to sort out a mess, she thought. The trouble is, you cannot trust other people to do it.

As she drove home to her flat, where she lived alone, Ann thought of the little old lady whose husband had suddenly dropped down dead that day, and who would be at home, alone. Suddenly, Ann began to cry for this woman and for herself. All the cars hooting reminded her that the lights had turned to green, and she mouthed a rude comment to the nearest driver. 'What's happening to me?' she thought. 'My mother would be horrified at what I have just said. It's this city, it's the job. I just need a holiday.'

Ann rang in the following day, to say she was ill with a migraine. She was irritated because the receiver of the call had remarked that Ann was getting lots of short periods of illness. The next day she was not well, but went to work because she felt guilty. Within a few hours she felt quite bright and engrossed in some routine, straightforward tasks like doing dressings and bandages — nothing too demanding.

A call came from ambulance control. A mother and child were being brought from a house fire. Neither was breathing. Ann felt panic. Why didn't this happen yesterday? Why does it always happen when I'm here? I have had too many of these bad ones to deal with. I wish I could just run away, she thought. Her thoughts were interrupted by a voice saying:

'Ann, the police have just rung. They have found the husband/father of the house fire victims at work. They are bringing him in now. Do you want to speak to him?'

Activity 8B

Give some formal and informal responses to Ann's plight.

REFERENCES

Atkins J, Piazza D 1987 Personality types of emergency nurses. Journal of Emergency Nursing 13(1):33–37
Bailey R D 1985 Coping with stress in caring. Blackwell Scientific, Oxford
Brunt C 1984 A very stressful place. Nursing Times 80(7):28–32
Burnard P 1987 Developing skills as a group facilitator. Professional Nurse 3:1
Burns A K, Kirilloff L H, Close J M 1983 Sources of stress and satisfaction in emergency nursing. Journal of Emergency Nursing 4(9):329–336
Caldwell M M 1976 Staff stress: what you can do about it. Journal of Emergency Nursing 2(2):21–23
Cannon W 1935 Stresses and strains of homeostasis. American Journal of Medical Sciences 189(1):1
Durham T W, McCammon S L, Allison E J 1985 The psychological impact of disaster on personnel. Annals of Emergency Medicine 14:7

Gendlin E T, Beebe J 1968 An experimental approach to group therapy. Journal of Research and Development in Education 1:19–29

Hare J, Pratt C C, Andrews D 1988 Predictors of burnout in professional nurses working in hospitals. International Journal of Nursing Studies 25(2):105–115

Hawley M P 1992 Sources of stress for emergency nurses in four urban Canadian emergency departments. Journal of Emergency Nursing 18(3):211–216

Keller K L 1990 The management of stress and prevention of burnout in emergency nurses. Journal of Emergency Nursing 2(16):90–95

Kolb L C 1986 Post-traumatic stress disorder in Vietnam veterans. New England Journal of Medicine 314(10):641–642

Lazarus R S 1966 Psychological stress and the coping process. McGraw Hill, New York

Lazarus R S, Folkman S 1984 Stress, appraisal and coping. Springer, New York

Levins S, Weinberg J, Ursin H 1978 Psychology of stress: a study of coping mechanisms. Academic Press, New York

McKechnie R 1993 Earwitness to disaster. Journal of Accident & Emergency Nursing 1(3):149–153

Mahoney B S 1991 The extent, nature and response to victimization of emergency nurses. Journal of Emergency Nursing 17(5):282–294

Manley K 1986 The dying patient in the intensive care unit — the problems. Care of the Critically Ill 2:4

Melia K M, Boyd K M 1994 Nursing ethics, 3rd edn. Churchill Livingstone, Edinburgh

Mitchell J T 1983 When disaster strikes: the critical incident stress debriefing process. Journal of Emergency Services, January, 122–127

Phipps L 1988 Stress among doctors and nurses in the emergency department of a general hospital. Canadian Medical Association Journal 4(139):375–376

Pot-Mees C 1987 Beating the burnout. Nursing Times 83:30

Selye H 1976 The stress of life, revised edn. McGraw Hill, New York

Wolfe H 1950 Life stress and bodily diseases. Williams & Wilkins, Baltimore

Woodruff I 1989 A report on staff reaction at Mayday University Hospital, following the major incident of the Purley train crash. British Journal of Accident and Emergency Medicine 4:2

Wright B 1989 Critical incidents. Nursing Times 83:19

Wright B 1992 Communication skills. Churchill Livingstone, Edinburgh

9

Holistic care

Underlying my philosophy of care and intervention in crisis situations is an holistic approach. I value the way this enables me to meet and know my clients better. I'd like to end the book with an outline of these holistic principles.

HOLISTIC PRINCIPLES

The principles are established to provide a framework that will enhance the carer/client relationship in many settings. The focus is on the following five human dimensions:

1. Physical
2. Emotional
3. Intellectual
4. Social
5. Spiritual.

This approach to treatment or therapy, developed by Herbert Otto in the early 1970s, may be used by all therapists regardless of their theoretical orientation. Despite the many approaches and areas of focus, holism makes assumptions that are common to all people. Holism recognizes that everyone has unrealized potential, that is best developed through self-responsibility and self-help.

People who have been affected by a sudden death will talk about a loss of control over their lives and about powerlessness or helplessness. One of our goals should be to help people regain control and power whilst giving them the freedom and space to express the pain of death.

Holism looks at the difficulties of being human and is concerned about the individual's existence. There is a premise that inner experience provides people with insights or their own sense of meaning and purpose, and that individuals make choices throughout life for which they are personally responsible. Within an holistic framework each person is considered unique.

Sudden death is a major health care issue, and can result in ill health as we have already discussed. Otto (1975) pointed out that all people seek good health; symptoms are expressions of need and motivate the person to seek help. What the sudden death means for an individual at the immediate time and later is always a major issue. Emphasis is put on life style and life goals, when working with the belief system and the meaning of life as seen by the individual person. Holism is clearly relevant in health care.

An holistic framework suggests opportunities to help individuals manage or cope with the crisis event. The five dimensions of holism can be applied to issues in the immediate and long-term care of the suddenly bereaved.

Physical dimension

People will describe how they react physically to certain stressful situations. Worry, for example, gives 'butterflies' or 'a knot in the stomach'. Some people experience a rapid heart beat, sweat or feel cold. The stress of a sudden death can also alter our bodies, and this in turn affects body image. In describing the impact of a sudden death, people will often ask:

'What is happening to me?'
or
'What has happened to me?'

They will perceive changes, some of which are clearly changes of body image — appearance, structure, size and shape. Some will describe themselves shrinking or carrying a heavy burden which bends them. Restlessness, fatigue, sleeplessness and vulnerability lead to feelings of physical weakness. Threats to body image are stressful because the ability to relate in meaningful ways to others often depends on our view of our image. Self-esteem or worth is closely interwoven with body image.

Emotional dimension

Stressors produce emotions that generate physiological responses. How we view our coping capacity is often related to the intensity of our feelings or emotions. We all experience responses, for example, laughing, crying, fear, trust, being full of hope and strength. The more unhealthy responses of hurt, guilt, resentment and helplessness cause us problems.

Absolute emotional health or illness is not easily defined. Emotional health is a process that evolves from emotional needs being met and a willingness to recognize and accept feelings, and perhaps use the energy generated positively. Emotional health has close links with acceptance of oneself and harmony with that self. On the emotional spectrum we respond to change in ways that are either healthy or unhealthy. The intensity and duration of the emotions depend on where we are on that continuum, and on our ability to satisfy our needs and experience, and to handle our feelings.

Intellectual dimension

The complex process of sensation or perception employs the central nervous system, which needs to be healthy and efficient. Memory, learning, cognitive and expressive functions are necessary components of our intellectual dimension. Someone who is healthy will function in these areas more effectively than someone who is not. Recent and past events, and our memory of them, help us to give current events meaning, and to understand them and perhaps increase our ability to cope. Defects of memory can affect our ability to understand relationships and events.

In the immediate impact of sudden death, and in the long term perplexity and work concerning its meaning, much thought and concentration will be needed. An elderly woman suffering from recent memory loss or forgetfulness whose husband has died suddenly may well have difficulty understanding the sequence of events around the death. This can cause her untold distress in taking in what happened and will require a protracted counselling process to clarify the details. Her need to examine the details is no less than anyone else's but her problems will frustrate her and make her angry. Losing flow of thought through cognitive difficulties causes great difficulties in managing the death in the long term.

Difficulties for the old and confused, and people with mental illness and handicap, are particular examples of problems in this dimension. Healthy individuals are capable of using expressive function to convey ideas and feelings; ill health may prevent this. So a stressor in the intellectual dimension may be any problem that prevents receptive function, memory, learning, expressive or cognitive functioning.

Social dimension

Many events in individuals' lives can contribute to social stress. Responses to social stress are determined by cultural values, past experiences in similar conditions, and the ability to cope with and understand the system. Relationships with support and nurturing may be found in the family network or may have to be sought in other areas, such as work, or from close friends. Our position or social class within the system may give us strength or stature, or a role; or it may not.

Social isolation, poverty, unemployment and marital or family difficulties cause problems if we have depended on these particular social dimensions for support. If we do not develop other social support systems when we are confronted with stress within our familiar system, we may not cope. Social interaction, which is the basis of social relationships, can give the right kind of stimulation towards recovery. It prevents isolation and encourages thought and growth. On the other hand, too much interaction is a violation of personal space and an infringement on our lives.

Much of the social dimension relates to perceived role. This may be apparent when the social structure makes conflicting or impossible demands on us, perhaps demands that conflict with our value system or roles that are ambiguous. Some roles conflict with each other and some, because of lack of preparation or training, make us feel incompetent. Full use of personal or professional resources is required for adequate performance of a role.

Some roles are temporary, others are imposed on us. In sudden death, this may mean all the aforementioned changes in the social dimension plus changes in sexual role and identity. The social dimension of sudden death requires a high level of adaptation and this produces severe stress.

Spiritual dimension

When people have to give a lot of attention and time to sorting out conflict that does not fit in with their belief system, the conflict becomes very stressful. The inability to meet spiritual needs adequately, because of the conflict, leaves them in a kind of vacuum. This challenge to the individual's beliefs attacks values and the individual is left in an unclear and ambiguous life position.

Our philosophy on life may have clarified our goals and values, leaving us free to follow our chosen path or direction. In turn, this decisive response will have confirmed our commitment to the chosen philosophy. Sudden death may question all this. Sudden death may indicate we got it wrong — we have failed because we did not reach the required standard. The wish to undo wrongs, to relive lives, expressions of shame and remorse, may become painfully apparent as suddenly as the death.

Spiritually healthy people have found reasons that give meaning to their existence: perhaps religion, or a relationship with nature and the universe. Some people have non-spiritual goals, such as money. Whatever the source of this meaning, it gives people a sense of hope and the ability to overcome adversity. Lack of purpose and life without meaning leads to despair and feelings of being useless or abandoned.

In periods of intense suffering people question the meaning of life and doubt their ability to overcome adversity. They question the value of the belief system they have or had. Eventually these feelings can lead to withdrawal and an overwhelming feeling of not being able to invest any more energy in seeking answers. They are stuck with the outcome and have a sense of resignation to suffering. At the time of sudden death, much time and energy has to be spent on these issues.

In the holistic philosophy each person is seen as multidimensional, with the five dimensions — physical, emotional, intellectual, social and spiritual — being in a continuing interaction with each other. The physical dimension involves everything that interacts with the body from without and within. The physiological and affective states, including motor mechanisms and the feelings that are involved, are included in the second area, the emotional dimension. The intellectual dimension covers receptive function, memory, learning and cognition. How we express this is also a function of the intellectual dimension. The social dimension involves social interaction and relationships as well as aspects of culture and the social systems. Finally, the spiritual dimension explores how people develop their understanding of the meaning of life, and how this will transcend or overcome various life difficulties.

These five major concepts, the basis of holistic philosophy, can be helpful in exploring responses to sudden death. Care should encompass looking into the immediate and long-term needs in all these dimensions. They offer a structured way of examining all components of the loss and identifying the areas that are being avoided. The important thing to remember though is that the holistic philosophy attributes individuals with the ultimate responsibility for what they will do with the insights gained from looking at each dimension. This focus of control is very important to people who have lost control or feel 'out of control'. The aim is for the individual who has lost someone, who is suddenly bereaved, to regain active participation and contribute to his own health status.

The five dimensions of a person are also useful in helping carers to re-evaluate themselves, particularly those who work with sudden death and other disastrous events. How we perceive this work impacting on us as carers is part of the process of caring for ourselves.

Activity 9A

Consider each of the five dimensions of a person. Now think about your experiences, either personally or with clients, involving sudden death. Write down the 'gains' and 'losses' you experienced in each dimension.

REFERENCE

Otto H 1975 Holistic therapy. In: Harper R (ed) The new psychotherapies. Prentice Hall, New Jersey

Conclusion

One difficulty in working with sudden death must be the awareness of its strength, enormity and complexity. Many people will have pondered what they would do if it happened to them, but then quickly decided that this is an exercise to be avoided. Perhaps we cannot live life to the full if we acknowledge the thought that a loved one can be taken from us suddenly. Perhaps there is little use in giving it any thought? If it happens, well, then we have to deal with it. So our ambivalent feelings towards sudden death present another difficulty in working with it — the problems become ours as well as our client's. 'What can we do about it?' is the question posed by a sudden death, but an underlying instinct is also to keep away from it.

The shock and disbelief of sudden death have much more impact than does an anticipated death. In his study of young widows/widowers in the Harvard Bereavement Study, Parkes (1975) was able to identify that in sudden death, there was clearly a more emotionally disturbed response. The disturbance persisted throughout the first year of bereavement. Another study (Lundin 1984), which followed up significant relatives 8 years after a death, found that where death was unexpected, feelings of remorse, self-reproach and distress were more marked than in those who had experienced an anticipated death.

Some sudden deaths produce even more problems than others. Sudden infant death syndrome (SIDS) or cot deaths lead to some very serious difficulties in the grieving process. I have seen several parents who have described themselves as being 'stuck' with some pain or difficulty. This standstill, or inability to leave some painful focus, can be with them for years.

Raphael (1984) describes the relentless search for the cause of death. Parents blame each other, and the role of the police and ensuing enquiries produce defensiveness and misunderstanding. Peppers & Knapp (1980) suggest that for most mothers the grief remains with them for the rest of their lives. They do not say it is persistently present but call it 'shadow grief,' describing it as a recurrent intrusion that casts a shadow across life. It is a transient reminder that, on occasions, produces a painful memory of loss and can shut out the joy of the present.

Whilst you would expect the death of a child to be especially problematical, where the death was anticipated the parents do not show more psychiatric symptoms than would be expected in any other kind of death. A study by Shanfield et al (1986) showed that in the anticipated death of a child, half of the parents reported a sense of personal growth and a great degree of intimacy with the rest of the family. Far worse outcomes were reported where the cause of death of the child was a road traffic accident. The difficulties were more marked for the mother than the father.

Wordon (1991) describes anticipatory grief as that occurring before the actual loss. Many deaths occur with some warning, and during this period of anticipation, the survivor begins some of the tasks of mourning, and begins to experience some of the grief. Wordon goes on to describe how, in sudden death, the prolonged grieving can produce resentment which leads to guilt. Anticipatory grief work may well have a better outcome, if the one who knows what the end result will be does not deny or suppress this knowledge. If the impending death is kept secret to avoid upsetting the dying person or other family members, the point of death can have all the hallmarks of a sudden death.

Death by suicide has, in my experience of counselling, resulted in some extremely difficult issues and must produce some very poor outcomes. The same applies to deaths by violence. Sudden death in these cases is not only a violation of the ones left behind but also a violation of their belief in life itself.

Sudden death, as we know from the experience of others, has the capacity to leave people damaged or to result in a prolonged and painful grieving process. The lack of time or preparation for the death leaves so much unfinished. This in turn leads to a double kind of grief — grief for what is lost and grief for what might have been.

There will usually be areas in the relationship that have been unrealized, areas that had greater potential. There will be unresolved emotional issues where, if there had been warning about potential loss, validation of feelings and confirmation of strengths in the relationship could have been given. The grief for themselves, and what might have been, is therefore inevitably an issue to discuss with bereaved clients. Grief for the deceased, what he has missed, his lack of time, and the injustice of this, compounds 'what might have been' for the bereaved:

'He was young and vital, so full of life. He never knew what it was like to fall in love or be a father.'

The many faces of sudden death demand great concentration and energy. What is lost and what might have been are just two of the issues that must be discussed. All the issues involved are very time-consuming to deal with, and use up a lot of energy. Some bereaved people describe themselves as being fed up with the whole thing, and lack the commitment to focus on or continue to work on the problem. They want answers, and in their search often come to an abrupt halt, holding up the process of grieving or prolonging it. The grief process becomes drawn out, imponderable and overwhelming.

When this happens it takes some effort, patience, skill and determination on the part of a counsellor to work with it. The counsellor must discover what stage this person has reached in his grief, and endeavour to make it manageable for him. We need to examine ways of breaking grief down into manageable components in the immediate and the long term. The suggestions in Chapter 1 are not blueprints for achieving clear and unequivocal outcomes, but may help make sudden death manageable by decreasing its impact and potential to damage.

Preventative medicine and its value in our health care system is another topic to consider with respect to the impact of sudden death. Glick et al (1974) demonstrate clearly how people with grief responses may present it in the (to them) more acceptable form of illness. Many of the young widows in Glick's study had increased visits to doctors within the first year of loss, with upper respiratory tract infections or gynaecological problems. This group, compared with a control group, had a higher incidence of these problems.

In our Accident & Emergency Department, I have noticed that many people with unresolved loss present with vague chest pains and panic attacks. Preventative medicine is low down on the list of health care priorities. Effective and committed intervention at the time of sudden death and afterwards could, however, greatly reduce the incidence of illness and injury to the bereaved resulting from this crisis. Raphael (1980) demonstrates how specific programmes for high-risk groups can effectively intervene. She discusses (Raphael 1984) how intervention is important both on impact and over time, in helping people come to terms with their loss.

REFERENCES

Glick I O, Weiss R S, Parkes C M 1974 The first year of bereavement. John Wiley, New York
Lundin T 1984 Morbidity following sudden and unexpected bereavement. British Journal of Psychiatry 144:84–88
Parkes C M 1975 Bereavement studies of grief in adult life, 2nd edn. Penguin, Harmondsworth
Peppers L G, Knapp R J 1980 Motherhood and mourning. Praeger, New York
Raphael B 1980 Primary prevention — fact or fiction? Australian and New Zealand Journal of Psychiatry 14:163–174
Raphael B 1984 The anatomy of bereavement: a handbook for the caring professions. Hutchinson, London
Shanfield S B, Benjamin G A H, Swain B J 1986 Parents' responses to the death of adult children from accidents and cancer: a comparison. American Journal of Psychiatry 141(9):1092–1094
Wordon J W 1991 Grief counselling and grief therapy. 2nd edn. Tavistock, London

Useful addresses

The Compassionate Friends
53 North Street
Bristol BS3 1EN
Tel: 0117 953 9639 (helpline)
        0117 966 5202 (administration)
Offers support and help for people suffering the loss of a child.

CRITEC — Crisis Counselling, Training, Education, Support
Tel: 0113 292 6498
Fax: 0113 292 6470
Offers crisis counselling service, training, counselling education, and debriefing for those working with sudden death and disastrous events.

CRUSE — Bereavement Care
126 Sheen Road
Richmond
Surrey TW9 1UK
Tel: 0181 332 7227
A counselling service with branches all over the UK. They have a wide range of literature and run bereavement counselling courses nationwide.

Foundation for Study of Infant Deaths
35 Belgrave Square
London SW1X 8QB
Tel: 0171 235 1721 (24-hour helpline)
        0171 235 0965 (general enquiries)
Advice and counselling for newly bereaved parents. Sponsors research and a wide range of literature for the caring professions.

Scottish Cot Death Trust
Royal Hospital for Sick Children
Yorkhill
Glasgow G3 8SJ
Tel: 0141 357 3946
Advice and counselling for newly bereaved parents. Sponsors research and a wide range of literature for the caring professions.

The Miscarriage Association
c/o Clayton Hospital
Northgate, Wakefield WF1 3JS
Tel: 01924 200 799
Support groups nationwide.

SANDS — Stillbirth and Neonatal Death Society
28 Portland Place
London W1N 4DE
Tel: 0171 436 5881
Information and support to bereaved parents, nationwide.

The Laura Centre
4 Tower St
Leicester LE1 6WS
Tel: 0116 254 4341
Counselling for bereaved parents. A list of videos and publications useful
for bereaved parents or those caring for them.

British Association for Counselling
37a Sheep Street
Rugby, Warwickshire CV21 3BX
Tel: 0178 878 328/9
Publishes directories of accredited counsellors. Concerned with training of
counsellors in a variety of settings.

Gay Switchboard
BM Switchboard
London WC1N 3XX
Tel: 0171 837 7324
24-hour helpline for lesbians and gay men, who can be referred to their
bereavement project.

Jewish Bereavement Counselling Service
14 Chalgrove Gardens
London NW3 3PN
Tel: 0171 349 0839
Trained volunteer counsellors for bereaved people.

Child Bereavement Trust
1 Millside, Riverdale
Bourne End, Bucks SL8 SEB
Support and counselling for bereaved families. Videos and literature for
training of carers.

Institute of Family Therapy
43 New Cavendish Street
London W1M 7RG
Tel: 0171 935 1651
Free counselling to newly bereaved families through the Elizabeth Raven Memorial Fund.

National Association for Staff Support
9 Caradon Close
Woking
Surrey GU21 3DU
Tel: 0148 377 1599
Coordinates and develops staff support for all health care staff. Organizes conferences and workshops and produces literature.

Support After Termination of Abnormality
22 Upper Woburn Place
London WC1H 0EP
Support group run by women and couples who have experienced termination of pregnancy because of abnormality.

Index